A - Z OF DISABILITY

MARTIE McBRIDE

A - Z
— OF —
DISABILITY

Life and Challenges with

Chronic Pain

First Printing, 2025

Cover Design by Bojan Reković
Book Interior Design by VMC Art & Design, LLC

ISBN: 979-8-9885681-3-1
Library of Congress Control Number: 1-14942970891

Delucslife Media LLC
30 N Gould St #3819
Sheridan, WY 82801

Printed in USA

This book is dedicated to Shane Burch, M.D.
whose skill as a surgeon is only surpassed by his
compassion and courage. I am so thankful he
inspired me to write this book.

A NOTE FROM THE PUBLISHER

We are thrilled to present Martie McBride's new book "A-Z of Disability." This remarkable book is a beacon of hope and resilience, chronicling Martie's incredible journey through chronic pain and her triumph over adversity. At the young age of 29, Martie's life took a challenging turn, yet she emerged stronger, finding new purpose and joy. Her story is not just about survival, but about thriving, and she shares her unique insights on pain management and self-advocacy with warmth and wisdom. Martie's accomplishments as an artist, athlete, and scholar, combined with her personal experiences, provide a rich tapestry of knowledge for anyone navigating similar challenges. Her message is clear: happiness and fulfillment are within reach, no matter the obstacles. We invite you to join Martie on this transformative journey and discover how to communicate effectively, seek support, and embrace a life full of joy and purpose.

INTRODUCTION

W hen it comes to being a human, it can be so confusing, right? You have your men and your women, your sane and your insane, and you have your able-bodied and your disabled. Some of us would like to have chosen our sex, as witnessed by the transgender thing going on. Most of us would prefer to be sane rather than insane. Tragically, it is often difficult to tell the difference because it is not a physically obvious condition. I believe all of us would prefer to be sane rather than insane and able-bodied rather than disabled. Sadly, being human means being fallible and is obviously more complex than sex, sanity, or disability.

I think the main problem is trying to walk in someone else's shoes, and thereby understanding them. When you cannot walk, and someone else can, there is a disconnect because walking is an entitlement we often take for granted.

The other problem is not all disabled people look impaired, some have mild conditions while others have severe restrictions. Like the rest of us, there is an origin story we cannot fathom unless it is shared. This is where I come in.

Funny thing about this book, I had tried to start it on three separate occasions. My pain and disability credentials are a 47-year history with a genetic form of Arthritis. My resume reads: 17 surgeries – including 2 total knee replacements, 2 total hip replacements, a complete spinal fusion, and a shoulder replacement.

In 2014, I needed help with my back because I could hardly walk. I had an amazing spinal surgeon who performed three mobility-saving fusions on my spine. My entire skeletal back is reinforced with metal pins at every vertebra level. I cannot turn my head. I can nod a lackluster YES, but I am a girl who can't say NO. This amazing and skilled surgeon suggested I write a book about my experience because he admired how I dealt with the pain. I tried three times previously and failed. I think it was too raw in my recovery after my surgeries to compose a manual of the important aspects disabled people, and the people who love and care for them, need to know.

Nowhere in this book do I purport to have medical expertise, quite the opposite: I am the patient. Never has the word patient been more apropos, because patience, humor, and courage will help you survive. I also acknowledge there are different levels of disability, but I think the universal truth is: whether you are temporarily disabled or permanently, your life has been altered in unforeseen ways.

There is a parable about a person who finds themselves in a hole, they have tried desperately to get out of. A holy person walks by, and the person in the hole yells, "Please help me, your holiness, I am stuck in a hole and cannot get out." The holy person says, "Of course, I will cite an incantation and throw a prayer for you to recite." The person in the hole recites the prayer over and over again. Nothing.

A doctor walks by and the person in the hole yells out again.

"Doctor, I am stuck in this hole and cannot get out." The doctor throws down a prescription bottle and says, "Surely, this will help you. Take 2 pills every 4 hours, and your problem should go away." The person in the hole does as instructed, but no results. Still stuck.

Finally, a friend walks by. The person in the hole pleads, "Friend, please help me. I am stuck in this hole and cannot get out." The friend jumps into the hole. The shocked person in the hole cries out, "What have you done?" The friend says, "Don't worry. I have been here before and I know the way out."

So, this A-Z book is my attempt to describe what it is like to be in the confusing and often dark world of disability. Here is my attempt to share how I have battled and survived a disease for 47 years.

It is not a medical treatise, it is not an attempt at scholarly study, it is just my attempt to articulate my journey with pain, disability and multiple surgeries in the hope others can find comfort. Because it comes down to that, how can life become more comfortable? Comfort? Forget comfort, think bearable, manageable, and tolerable. These are the words that replace self-fulfillment, self-actualization, goal setting, and motivation – all those watchwords and ambitions of modern life must now take a back seat. In my case, it was a genetic form of Arthritis that felled an otherwise healthy 29-year-old woman. It is going to take a bit of time and explaining for you readers to understand.

A - Z
OF
DISABILITY

A

ABLEISM

Imagine two people walking into a restaurant. One is erect and moving freely in their body, let's call this person Able. Able is most likely excited about eating at the restaurant. Able doesn't have to think twice about how they are going to cross the room, what chair they can sit in, what foods will accommodate their dietary needs, how they are going to get to a bathroom, if necessary. In reality, they are able-bodied.

The other is somehow altered – perhaps a limp, perhaps they have a cane or crutches, perhaps they are in a wheelchair or using a walker – let's call that person Hobble. Hobble has a different set of thoughts than Able. Hobble is most likely excited about the restaurant, being with a friend, and eating food someone else has prepared. But Hobble is also concerned about how they will be received, how to navigate the room, what chair will be comfortable for them to sit in, or if they are in a wheelchair, is there enough space to cross the room without knocking into stuff, and will the table accommodate their chair?

If Hobble is a bit wobbly and has an uncertain gait, they are worrying about bumping into other people or objects. They are also worrying about the toilet accommodations, does this restaurant even have handicapped spaces or grab bars? A lot more is preoccupying Hobble's mind than having a relaxing time out with someone else preparing the food.

Now, let's talk about the other patrons in the restaurant. When Able and Hobble enter and are noticed, there will be, more often than not, judgment. We are humans and we notice differences. Able will be judged to be NORMAL, and Hobble ABNORMAL. Some patrons are warmly inclusive and accommodating – let's call them Kindred. Other patrons will have coldly harsh reactions, mostly feeling they are entitled to a meal out without having to look at any form of deformity - let's call them Priss.

The reality is that all of us will compute that Hobble has something WRONG with them. It doesn't have to be said, because it is seen. And in that reality of being different, it can become a very awkward space for able-bodied people to know how to act, what to say, or what to do.

Kindred will have empathy and concern, but unless they are used to dealing with people with disabilities, their behavior can often become anxious. How do I help? What should I do? Some will hit the notes just right: polite and helpful. But so often, they will become obsequious in their excessive concern for Hobble, making them feel even more out of place. Because that is the issue: Hobble cannot control their environment and would rather be part of the scene than that awkward oddity.

Priss will perceive Hobble as damaged goods, and will act oblivious to their presence, or actively annoyed. I have experienced both and prefer Kindred's concern. Even with a warm welcome, I want to meld into the scene, not to stick out and be obvious, but that is literally impossible. For me, not only do I walk with an awkward gait, I cannot turn my head. A noticeable defect, I would think. And this is where it gets even more complicated.

Does one ask what happened? Does one pretend nothing is amiss? I often realize part of that reticence to ask is polite, why bring up a sore subject? This is the dilemma Kindred contemplates – no hate, but concern.

I am guilty of this myself. I wasn't in a restaurant, but in a sauna. I have a lot of scars on my body – replaced knees, hips, spine, and shoulder result in a lot of scars. A lady came in who had an amputated leg and used a crutch to stabilize herself. I had noticed her swimming in the lap pool. Even with one leg, she could swim while I was relegated to the shallow exercise pool. I really wish I could have swam with her.

When she came into the sauna and sat down, she commented on my scars, very kindly. But I felt inadequate to ask about her missing leg. She seemed friendly and open, but I was internally ashamed because I am mobile despite my painful surgeries.

But hers was a life quite different from mine, and I didn't know how to broach the subject. That was many years ago, and I believe today I would ask, and we could talk about our struggles. But in that sauna and in that moment, my tongue was tied because I didn't know if I wanted to hear her story, and know her pain. Perhaps I was still too engaged in my own struggle. I don't think that lady took offense to my non-curiosity, but looking back, I would have liked to have known what had happened to her. Sometimes we can handle the truth, and sometimes it is too much to imagine.

What has brought Hobble to this point, what happened? Perhaps by inquiring, one might hear a story that is painful and agonizing, or maybe it is politeness. Why bring up the past? Really, who wants to go there? But Hobble carries their story into any room they enter. It is written all over their bodies.

That takes us to Priss, a horse of a different color. Priss marches through life righteously convinced of their own perfect invincibility. They perch on a higher loft than we. Although I think there are more Kindred people in the world than Prisses, the Prisses somehow make it all awful for Hobble and I think for Kindred, as well.

I have experienced the ugliness of Priss. I walk with an awkward gait. I cannot use a cane or walker because the strain on my neck, back, and shoulders would be too much for my frame to handle.

Therefore, I am an obvious target for the haters out there. I have had people point and stare and yell, even across the street, "YOU WALK FUNNY," and they don't mean haha funny, they mean you're a freak to them. This doesn't happen when I am out with friends or family, but it does happen. A very public politician even made fun of a disabled journalist on national TV, and to my knowledge, Meryl Streep was the only voice to point out the shameful behavior. Sadly, some people are shameless.

Some of my surgeries, when new, have very dramatic scar patterns, especially my complete spinal fusion. It looked like a zipper on my back for about a year, at first angry and red, then dark and noticeable, but the scar would eventually fade. My back was hidden under clothing and the most noticeable part was my neck.

One day, when my neck scars were still fresh from my cervical fusion, I was coming out of the pool after water exercise, and a man, who was the husband of a friend, felt compelled to point out my neck scars. He pointed at them and was almost shouting – "You have an ugly looking railroad track on your back, I would never let that happen to me." That's the point – it didn't happen to them, but rarely do they realize it MIGHT.

These are minor and rather benign encounters, but they cut into a Hobble's sense of well-being. Seriously, do you have to be so unkind?

When I am in a wheelchair being pushed by someone, I feel incredibly vulnerable. I wish I were capable of having an electric wheelchair that I could manipulate myself, but my lack of vision and the stiffness of my neck make it impossible to navigate in public.

So many times I have witnessed the kindness of strangers. But I have also experienced the derision and exclusion of the haters, and it can drive a person to stay home and not go out.

Another reaction might result in ignoring or somehow dismissing or belittling the disabled person. They might extend their sympathy or empathy or compassion to the erect person – my goodness, what a saint to step out with a disabled person.

Regardless of the reaction, the disabled person is, more often than not, seen as a weak or damaged individual. Something is WRONG with them. In truth, they are compromised in some way by their bodily function or appearance. So, getting beyond that point with them, neglecting or negating their physicality becomes an awkward issue.

Trust me, disabled people get it. We understood early on in

our odyssey with our bodily systems that we do not fit the definition of "normal", and for some reason that makes us sub-human.
A lesser being.

Ableism is defined as "a system of discrimination and prej-
udice against people with disabilities that is based on the idea
that people without disabilities are superior."

ACCESS

Nowhere are the playing fields more divergent for Able and
Hobble than when it comes to the freedom of going places.
Whether it is old buildings with only staircase entries, businesses or establishments on the second floor without elevators;
or businesses on the ground floor with no automatic doors or
a theater or sports arena where seating is a climb. So often,
ACCESS DENIED is the message we receive.

Think about it for a moment. When you are on your computer,
whizzing through the internet, and you are directed to a website
where you need special codes or instructions. You get the
ACCESS DENIED impediment. It may take you several tries to
crack the code, and then you enter. Or maybe, you accept your
bad luck and give up, probably with some frustration and maybe
some cursing at being denied entrance.

In the physical world, there are often places clearly marked
NO ENTRY, regardless of one's physicality. Like nuclear test

sites, operating rooms, or airport runways. Nobody goes there that isn't authorized.

Let's imagine Hobble is on their own. They are wheelchair bound, or use a walker, or don't have use of their arms. Hobble arrives at a destination only to discover there aren't doors that open automatically. Hopefully and quite commonly, a kind stranger will come along, see the dilemma, and assist. I wish that were a hundred percent guarantee, but sadly, if Hobble knows they can't enter easily, they will stop trying and go somewhere else.

When there is an older building or when I am in a city where buildings were built before electric doors and elevators, I am often denied access.

Many years ago, I was the new member of a very old and venerable women's club. The edifice it inhabits was built in the late 1800's. The building is graceful and elegant – a site for many weddings or special celebrations. But there were absolutely no ramps or elevators to enable disabled people to enter. I decided to raise money so they could adapt a space for a ramp. I even suggested this ramp could be in the back, unnoticed by most people, perhaps by the service delivery area. After I raised the money they informed me, "that isn't the look we are going for." Forget about having a wedding where your old granny cannot even enter the building, talk about a shock.

The truth was, it wasn't about the ramp, it was the people who needed to use it. This makes me very sad and angry because, let's be honest, I get that there is nothing attractive or sexy about walkers and canes and wheelchairs, and it might make other people face their own aging process or bring down the property values or something inane like that. This attitude saddens me beyond measure, because with our aging population, Disability will come to many of you, if not all of you, and I am hoping the people around you have compassion and an understanding of ACCESS.

My personal journey with NO ACCESS is nowhere more pronounced than in parking lots. For the past 20 years, I have had ambulatory issues, in other words, it is hard to walk. When I do get to go out, like a fun dinner or shopping, I will often be disappointed there are no handicap spaces. Let me explain, whenever I go out, there are rarely available handicap spaces – Costco, malls, the airport, physicians' offices, movie theaters, etc. We just take it as a given. Mind you, most of the folks I see exiting their vehicles do not have any noticeable sign of disability.

I know there are many disabilities that are not disfiguring or manifest in noticeable limps; however, I am well aware that family members often tell themselves they are making this mission FOR their handicapped loved one, but they themselves are not impaired. Or maybe they don't care and snagged a placard.

This need to be the closest car in the lot confounds me. I used to belong to a fitness center which perplexed me even more. If you want exercise, why insist on the closest parking spot? Is it your sense of entitlement and competitive victory that gives them a "one up" on us invalids? Quite simply, they are often depriving me of my opportunity to access where I am going.

The fitness center had a big parking lot, so it was not too inconveniencing. In other scenarios, my driver can deposit me in front of an establishment, but sometimes that is not even an option. So please, able-bodied people out there, please stop taking the handicap spaces of people who are physically impaired.

———

ARTHRITIS

For me, arthritis has been my nemesis for forty-seven years. I was 29 years old when I was struck with projectile vomiting so intense I had to be hospitalized. This was tricky, because I was also the single mother of a 7-year-old daughter. My brother dropped me at the door of the hospital, then went home to be with my daughter. Fortunately, I knew most of the doctors and hospital staff, because I had worked at that hospital.

The year was 1978 and there were no CT scans, and no MRI's. They couldn't stop the vomiting, so I was put in the CCU (Critical Care Unit) one step down from ICU (Intensive Care Unit). I would be there for three days throwing up. Finally, they diagnosed me with Degenerative Disc Disease (DDD), which is a form of Osteoarthritis. My neck had a degenerated disc pressing on the nerve controlling digestion.

That was the beginning of my transformation – a reverse Pinocchio effect. Over time, I was a real girl turned into a metallic cyborg which is: "a living organism with both biological and mechanical parts that enhance its abilities."

We like to think we live in modern times and have modern answers for ancient diseases, but I wonder if we are as advanced as we think. Arthritis is actually a prehistoric disease. Archeological digs have revealed arthritic conditions in skeletal remains of cave people, even mummies entombed in Egypt have shown evidence of the deformity. The word itself is a compound of ancient Greek – ARTHO for joint, and ITIS for inflammation.

The problem with arthritis is the word. Everybody has heard it, everybody thinks they know what it means when they age, but seriously, it is an illness that defies concrete definition. CAUSE we know – inflamed joints. EFFECT is the unknown because it is so individual. There are over 100 different types of arthritis. Twenty million people in our country are afflicted with one form or another, but not all forms are created equal. Actually, 70% of arthritic cases present in elderly people, over 60. That means 30% of the cases come to younger people, like me. Then there is Juvenile Arthritis, a heartbreak all its own. Some variations are more crippling, painful and destructive than others, but the general consensus seems to be, the earlier in life you get arthritis, you will get a more virulent and aggressive variety.

When I meet people who want to bond and find a common playing field, I become a bit concerned. Any pregnant person can understand, people will regale you with the stories they feel compelled to share.

Kindly intentioned people often wax on philosophically in an attempt to connect with me by relating their journey with arthritis – how their maiden aunt suffered for years, or how they themselves overcame it in an heroic effort. Rarely are they talking about the same form or variation of arthritis. The more notable varieties are Rheumatoid Arthritis (RA), Psoriatic Arthritis (PSA), and Osteoarthritis (OA) which is the umbrella term for Degenerative Joint Disease and Degenerative Disc Disease.

Early days in my dance with arthritis or Arthur, as I prefer to think of this disease, like an abusive partner who has had coercive control over me for 47 years, I was naïve about the impact it would have on my life.

Back in 1978, there wasn't a tremendous amount of support for people afflicted with either variation, but the diagnosis I got was Degenerative Disc Disease which is a painful form of Osteoarthritis. In fact, Osteoarthritis tops the pain charts in the world of arthritis. It is on the Top Ten list of most painful diseases.

But Rheumatoid Arthritis (RA) is an extremely painful auto-immune disease all on its own. I started with Osteoarthritis 47-years ago, but 15-years ago, I got a new traveler in my body. It was Psoriatic Arthritis which is closely associated with Rheumatoid Arthritis.

A dear friend, who was a stained-glass artist, was struck with RA in her mid- forties. Her hands became too crippled to work, so she had to change career paths. For me, I was the administrator of my own company, one that managed doctor's offices. I, too, had to change professions. It is a life-altering disease that can really wreak havoc with any future planning.

Unlike other highly publicized and deadly diseases, like some cancers or ALS, arthritis is unique and specific to different people. For some, it is a benign restriction, for others, it can be life-altering in unimaginable ways, a real game changer. No longer is my life about setting goals, accomplishing tasks, or completing bucket lists – my job is to endure. Arthur is the driver, and I am along for the ride. Remember, arthritis has been around since caveman times, so the journey will be rocky.

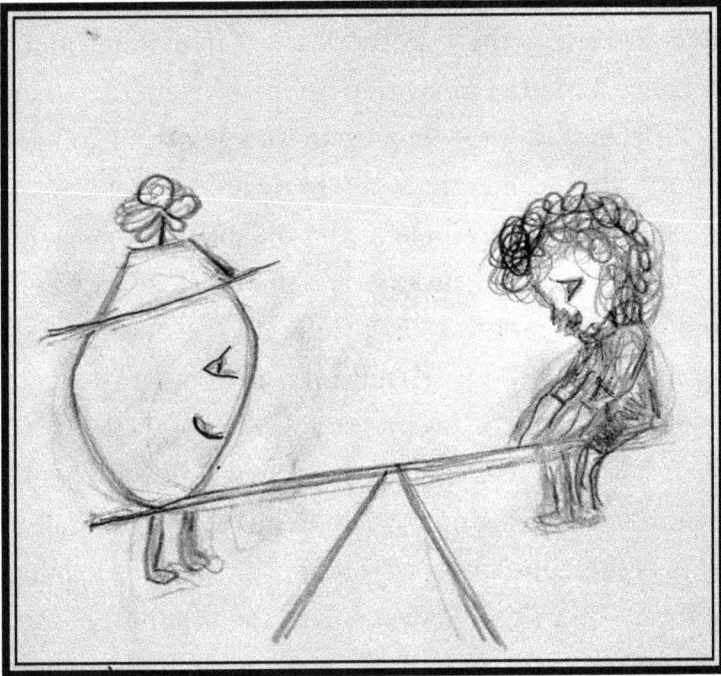

BALANCE

Balance is a critical component of modern life and there are two types, emotional balance and physical balance.

Emotional balance is a struggle for all of us – right/wrong – work/play – anger/joy – achievement/frustration. There are literally an endless variation of dichotomies we all must face.

For disabled people their work is taking care of their mind/

body – not much space for play. Physical therapy, massage therapy, infrared treatments, ablations, stimulating implants, and all the various medical regimens that can ameliorate the pain and discomfort replace the fun stuff.

The real comfort, for me, has come with water exercise or massage therapy – these activities are individual and rarely social. I once joined a Pain Group because I wanted to hang with fellow sufferers, to know how their struggle was going. Sadly, attendance was so erratic because disabled people with pain aren't the paralympic athletes, the disabled people with pain are the ones staying close to home, being close to where they can find comfort and feel safe. Being in the outer world, even joining with sympathetic friends and sufferers, rarely happens. This is not a club anyone wants to join.

When it comes to anger, I can only speak for myself. I am angry this disease was inflicted upon me. It was generated by an aunt I never met, but the story is that she was wheelchair-bound before forty. This would have been in the first half of the twentieth century. Modern medicine with joint replacements and spinal fusions has spared me her fate.

Yet, there are insults and agonies to be angry about – an insensitive comment, a difficulty getting into a car or doctor's office, all the physical restrictions I must encounter on the daily. Acceptance goes a long way in soothing myself. I did not cause it, I cannot control it, and I cannot change it. This is my fate. It sucks big time, but to be in a constant state of anger or agitation is not a recipe for peace and calm. I always try to meditate rather than agitate.

Finding joy when I am in high levels of pain is impossible,

one just needs to endure and survive. When the pain passes, I do rejoice that I survived another attack. But like a veteran warrior, I tire of the assaults. One day, when the BIG PAIN becomes incessant, I know I will lose the will to live. But for now, I endure.

The reason I endure is that I have a family who loves me very much, and I them. They have been on this long journey of replaced joints, endless tests and treatments, and frustrating recoveries.

When I had my cervical fusion, I could not be left alone for two weeks lest I choke to death with the inability to swallow and clear my throat. I needed constant care. One of my daughters would lie next to me in bed and when the terrible gagging and choking started, they would prop me to clear my airways, they took 8-hour shifts because it was a 24-hour issue. This is a terribly frightening experience for everyone involved. This is an example of the love and devotion my family gives me, and it gives me reason to endure all my suffering. I try to do it with grace and not be a royal pain in the ass, but it isn't easy when you deal with high levels of pain. (A subject under P.)

But make no mistake, if you are a disabled person, it takes the entire household to accept the alterations in your combined universe. There may be ramps into the house, there may be ergonomic seats in every room, there may be handicapped toilets and showers, a hospital type of bed to change elevations – maybe more, I just name a few that come to mind. Everyone now lives in your new reality, and for some, that is not the look they are comfortable with. You find out real fast the true colors of people in your life.

The hardest balance for me to find is between achievement and frustration. What was once an assured trajectory of graduate school and occupation was now a hall of mirrors. Constantly looking at my own distortions. Not having any energy to engage in an enterprise other than getting through the day.

Balance also means the physical ability to balance oneself. To be able to stand on one foot. This sounds silly, I'm thinking, to most folks, but it is a critical element for the disabled and the elderly. Balance is critical for a smooth walking gait; it also reduces the risks of falling.

This is where Humpty Dumpty comes into focus. He was a good egg, just minding his own business sitting on a wall, and he lost his balance – the rest is history. Because sometimes this is the way it all happens – cracking all at once. But for some, it is a slow burn of being eaten alive by incessant cartilage munchers, as I refer to my personal invaders.

This is where my story comes into focus. For me, it was not a fall off the wall, but I was blameless. Not running marathons, not stressing my body to its limits. I was just a single mom who ran her own business.

Imagine, if you can, being 29 years old, at the top of my game. The year was 1978 and I was six months shy of 30. For me, one of the important definitions I had of myself was an athlete. Athletics had helped me survive a toxic and dysfunctional family by giving me an outlet to belong to a group and it helped me gain tremendous self-esteem.

Every sport I could find to help me escape the house as much as possible was the one I played. Fortunately, I was good at it. Captain, usually, of any team I joined. I loved all sports – swimming, tennis, and horseback riding were my favorites. For me, time was wasted inside – I gloried in the outdoors. I was the kid you had to call in from the playground. First out in the morning, and last to leave at the end of the day.

Nowadays, I often struggle to go outside. There is always the issue of falling. I still get in the pool – but instead of long swims, I do water exercise. That brings us to physical balance. It was at water exercise where I regained my lost sense of balance. I could stand on one foot in the water, and finally made the transition to land. The water is so forgiving. Joints and muscles that drag on land can be buoyant in the water. Don't underestimate the need to balance on one foot. It helps with walking, sitting, and climbing stairs.

I was particularly keen to climb stairs. I had not been able to do so for about 10 years, but I wanted to visit my daughter whose house has five flights of them. It took me four months of physical therapy and six months of aching legs which felt like I was the Little Mermaid trying to transition to being human. Fortunately, I succeeded and was able to conquer that inadequacy. I could climb stairs. Not elegantly, but I got there. If you are holding out for graceful and effortless walking or climbing, think again. Those days are gone and it is unlikely they will return.

BEDRIDDEN

There is a trick to being a bed jockey, as I prefer to call it, instead of bedridden. Or bed confined. Or bed bound. It is a tricky space to master. For me, I was bedridden five years BEFORE my transformative surgeries, and then another five years AFTER recovering from 7 surgeries.

Remember I am a single mother. The family members I had were my teenage daughters. It was also the time when Amazon wasn't in full stride, but there was a meal delivery service I discovered – one the movie stars used on their travels. There are work-arounds, but you must embrace them and not drain your loved ones too much.

My bed is where all things nurturing are – a comfortable mattress, the optimal amount of pillows and supports. It is my nest. It has also housed me in times of great distress. Recovering from 17 surgeries is quite a test of one's ability to stay optimistic. I still spend a massive amount of time in my bed. Having a metal spine doesn't make for comfort in sitting in a chair or a car or an airplane. My bed comforts me.

I make my bed beautiful – the right cotton sheets are something you need to consider, because if you have the pain levels I do, you will sweat. Pain makes you sweat, sort of like menopause that never goes away. For you gentlemen out there, this will give you a taste of what most women endure. I also have artwork and plants that give me pleasure. The atmospherics are important.

I am not Maria from The Sound of Music. I do have favorite things, but I cannot sing. My comforts are mostly music and listening to podcasts. Sadly, reading a book is not an easy option, but can be accomplished with a great deal of preparation and large fonts on my e-book. I used to read a few books a week, but now I am lucky to read one of my e-books in a month.

So, being ever resilient, I try to focus on the world of imagination rather than the world of pain. That balance is an incredibly difficult achievement, but if you persist you, too, can overcome obstacles that want to drag you into despair. For me, I can no longer watch cable news or cable television – the ads alone make me want to jump out of a window. The feeble and immobile are constantly on parade in commercials. What a sick sort of nation are we?

I prefer streaming networks with no commercials, but I find they are now nickel-and-diming me because they used to be commercial-free but now, there are sneaky add-on costs.

BODY IMAGE

Image is everything, right? So in my case, I was 29 years old, and at the top of my game. In graduate school while I was writing my thesis for a Masters in Business Administration, I conceived of an idea to manage doctors' offices. I had previously worked in the Emergency Room managing the ER doctor's corporation. I had also worked for the Medical Staff Secretary and knew most of the doctors in town because I had, for several years, been the screener and verifier for physician's hospital privileges. Remember, these were pre-computer days.

That background gave me a launch pad for my business. The basic thesis was that doctors were well trained in

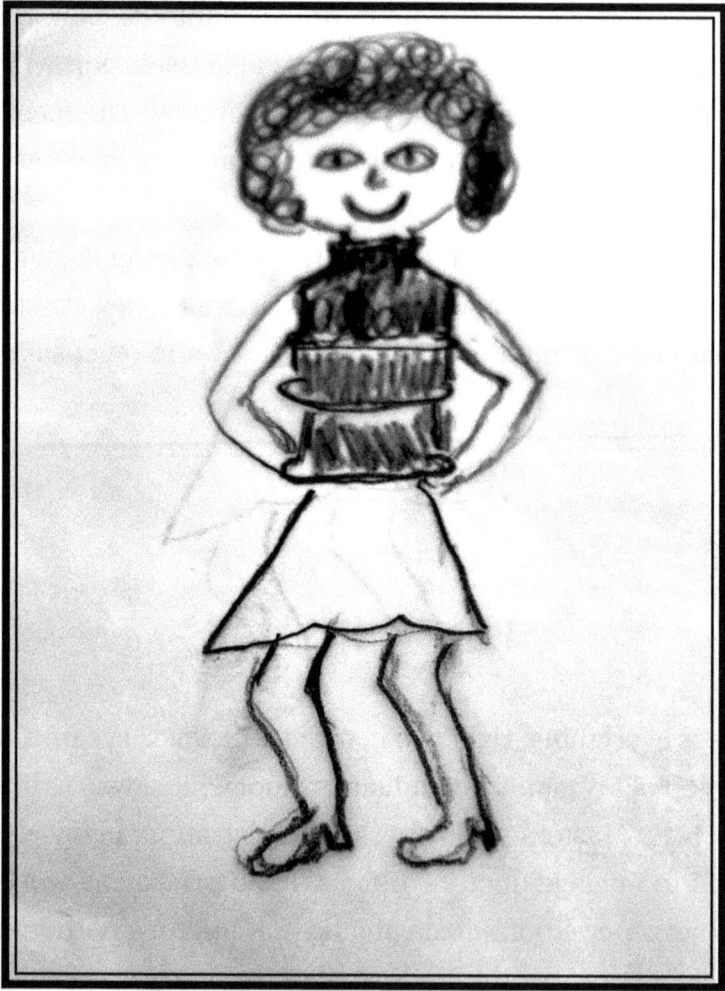

whatever medical practice they had studied, but were, quite often, ill-trained to manage a business. The mega groups of doctors we have today weren't in place in the town where I lived, so a newly qualified doctor would set up his own practice, usually with his wife as the receptionist or a nurse, sometimes the wife was both nurse and office help. Most physicians who enter the real world to practice medicine have accumulated a mountain of debt to get the white jacket and the initials after their name.

I have such admiration for the work and personal sacrifice it takes to become a physician.

The premise of my company, Physicians Management Services, was I would hire, fire, and supervise all the doctor's employees, they would be part of my company. I quickly established a reputation for fixing troubled offices with better cash flow and more efficiency. If I had a woman (all my employees were women, a sign of the times – not many male nurses or office workers) who was an exceptional receptionist, she could have a hope for promotion and advancement. At the height of my success, I had fourteen physicians to manage and 28 employees to wrangle, and a household to run all by myself, which had a child present.

At that time, it was mandated that if you ran a small business which applied to physicians and their practice, you needed to give your employees the same benefits which included health insurance and any retirement plan opportunities. In those days, doctors didn't really need much health insurance because there was a reciprocal agreement that there was a no charge policy for other physicians and their families. So, my business gave my employees, 28 women, a decent health insurance plan, and provided mental health days. My business was going well and I could charge $150 an hour (about $700 an hour in today's dollars) to consult. I didn't get too many of those jobs and found them frustrating. It is one thing to have the time to fix a troubled office system, but difficult to succinctly prescribe a solution. I did it well enough, I guess, because I did a fair number of consulting jobs. My main focus was my physicians and employees.

When I got struck with the ugly stick that is arthritis, I was blindsided. I don't know that anyone is particularly prepared for this kind of news, but I needed to change my self-image. My size five body was encased in a plastic neck brace for six months, and later I would have all sorts of casts, crutches, braces, and support systems to keep me mobile.

I was no longer in the fast lane. I was in the slow-as-you-go lane. I became The Cripple. Of course, I didn't see myself that way, but it is almost impossible to ignore the different ways people now treated me.

Prior to my hospitalization and diagnosis, I was Alpha Woman, an ascending entrepreneur, who had conceived a revolutionary way for doctors to run their offices. To this day, I believe companies have taken this space and run with it. In my day, prior to 1978, it was a fledgling concept. I couldn't even convince my doctor clients about using computers. It was the wave of the future. Of course, in hindsight, we get that, but then computer technology, too, was a fledgling industry that hadn't taken over the world.

That is my personal moment of adjustment. But consider some more famous figures who had challenges to their self-image. I am thinking of Mohammed Ali and Michael J. Fox in this category. As much as I admired Ali's athleticism, I think his humanitarian image is what endures. He did not shrink from his Parkinson's. He bravely carried on. Didn't withdraw.

And there aren't enough accolades in the English language to describe the admiration I have for Michael J. Fox. We, of a certain age, remember his youthful and charming exuberance. Now, we see his courage and commitment to healing and coping with an incredibly devastating disease. He carried on, despite his altered body image. For that, I believe he has made his greatest impact.

One of my saddest memories is of Rosalind Russell, who was a model and a movie star of the 1930's and 1970's. She often starred with Cary Grant, and was Auntie Mame on Broadway and in the movies. She portrayed professional women who were gutsy and not sex symbols, although she was beautiful enough to be one. She was nominated four times for best Actress at the Oscars.

I used to love watching her – she had a free-spirited approach to life, and I loved her in Auntie Mame. Unbeknownst to the general public, she also had Rheumatoid Arthritis, a condition she contracted in 1969, after her acting career had diminished. I was introduced to her disease when she came on stage during the Academy Awards, perhaps being honored for a lifetime achievement award, I don't remember and can't find any internet references. She was frail and needed a walker or a cane, I can't remember which. When she came on stage, the entire audience gasped and went silent. She shrugged and said something like, "You're not having it." And she turned around and walked off stage. It was an awkward moment, but it is a scene I have replayed in my head many times over the years. As an actress, appearance is everything, but for me, I had truly loved her spunky attitude, and it disappointed me she was so ill received.

Other notable celebrities with Rheumatoid Arthritis are tennis players Caroline Wozniacki and Danielle Collins; football player Terry Bradshaw; Kathleen Turner, actress; and Paula Abdul, the dancer and performer.

Linda Ronstadt was another poignant public figure whose life was interrupted by disease. Originally, it was thought she had Parkinson's – the symptoms started in 2002 but became crippling in 2012. Later the diagnosis became Progressive Supranuclear Palsy, which manifests in similar symptoms to Parkinson's.

I admire her immensely because she doesn't shrink from interviews, she has issues with her incredibly beautiful voice and cannot sing any more, but her spirit shines through like a beacon. Her will to be seen and to be heard has always inspired me.

Another notable celebrity with a degenerative disease was Annette Funicello, the bouncy Mouseketeer from my childhood. She had Multiple Sclerosis and tried to work, until the disease overcame her. I remember hearing murmurings about her, but when I looked her story up to research this book, I was amazed how long she truly did carry on despite her disease. She went quietly, as I recall. Not much attention is given to a celebrity once they can no longer entertain us.

Of course, there is more going on with these people than loss of body image – there is also a loss of career and doing what they loved. It's not like you suddenly developed a rash and you carry on, these diseases are painful and debilitating.

It takes courage to remain in the harsh gaze of the public eye. There might be gestures of acceptance, but the reality of being part of the scene in the way you were before is mitigated even if you are able to carry on. Your main job now is to manage pain and disease, not to carry on as if nothing is going on.

C

CARETAKER

When I first started writing this book, I thought I would comprise a list of Do's and Don'ts – ten things to do for arthritis, that sort of thing. But the list got unwieldy, and I am not really good at chronological order, as you can tell I jump around. However, had I chosen that approach, the first maxim would be:

BE NICE TO THE PEOPLE TAKING CARE OF YOU

Remember, your life has changed forever, but so has your family's. Gone are the fun outings – no more relaxed and spontaneous trips to the park, to the movies, to museums, to the mall, to the store – the myriad of events that make up family life. Now, it is trips to the doctor, the hospital, x-ray, physical therapy, lab tests, emergency rooms. All these fun events have been replaced by the nightmare that is Disability.

Remember, it is your nightmare. All you can do is hope they will be along for the ride. But in no way is it their fault. Your frustration with life's sour grapes should not allow you to make a toxic wine for your loved ones. Your job now is to manage your condition. If it happens to be a very painful condition, like mine, then it will become that much more difficult.

The problem is synthesizing what is happening to you and

separating it from expecting those around you to FIX it. They can only engage with you. Hopefully, if you aren't so negative, they will want to.

I am reminded of an incident while I was at a doctor's appointment sitting in the waiting room. A man came in with a harried woman trailing behind him. He had an aura of anger about him, and the aura spread like wildfire in the waiting room. He started cursing the poor woman, "You f*****g moron, you never do anything right," – that sort of thing. I have no idea if she was his wife or his caretaker, but it became really uncomfortable to be in the room with him going off. I went to the bathroom hoping he would disappear, but when I returned, he was still going at it – berating this woman incessantly.

I spoke up because I rarely suffer in silence and I said, "You are making it very uncomfortable to be in the same room because of your unpleasant attitude." He snapped back, "I am sick." And I replied, "You are not the only one." At that moment, I was called into the exam room. He was gone when I came out, but I will always count my blessings that I don't know that man.

I get the frustration of pain and disability and the loss of confidence in your own body. I get that if you are dealing with a disease or injury, you are trying to engage with your own feelings, but please try to sort through your issues because you need positive people around you, not people afraid of your rage.

As a psychologist, that is my training. What are you feeling? Anger? Frustration? Pain? – these top the list. The satisfaction of action is denied to you, so you must become a describer without becoming too macabre. The problem is, of course, the pain is written all over your face, and those who love you see it.

You have become a dependent person. Depending on your capacities, food will now be delivered to you, not prepared or purchased by you. I think mealtime can be an extremely uncomfortable time for the disabled. I am not fond of eating in bed, but sometimes it is unavoidable. I am really particular about my diet because being gluten-free and dairy-free does not make for quick and convenient take-away meals. If the caretaker ignores your needs or simply doesn't have the wherewithal to create healthy meals, you may feel even more miserable.

If you are head of a household, like I was, the challenges are monumental. I was a single mother through every surgery I had. My children were called to task at a very early age. Many a high school or college vacation was spent taking me to surgeries or to the doctors. Forget the embarrassment of having a dork of a mom drive around in a neck brace or having a car with handicapped license plates – forget those inconveniences.

I am talking about battles in the trenches. I am talking about the loss of a normal childhood. My oldest daughter lost her father to his troubled mind after the Vietnam War, my other two children lost their father to mental illness and cancer. Having a disabled mother has kept them in the medical loop of death, disease, and disability. I don't know many mothers or fathers who would choose that sort of childhood for their loved ones. Now you must not only deal with the frustration of your disease, but also the implicit impact it has on your family.

COMPASSION

This is a tricky subject. I am not sure you can teach compassion. Some see a disabled person and feel sympathy, others see a disabled person who is weak and should be eliminated from their sight. I am sure the elimination is not really what some of them are seeking, but the reality is, they don't want to LOOK AT IT.

During the early 1990s, my eldest daughter was at university in New York City. For some reason, the 90s seemed more forgiving. She was working on the American Disabilities Act, trying to make museums more accessible to disabled people. I think this was a universal effort, not just here in the United States.

Museums are magical and museums are a wonderful escape for everyone, but more so the disabled. The colors and shapes and statues and paintings remind us of our need for beauty. I am so pleased there was a concerted effort to include access for disabled people.

The matter of compassion is tricky because I am not sure a lot of people can see outside themselves to engage with other people's pain. I am remembering my sauna encounter with the one-legged woman. I wasn't cruel, I just didn't have a clue what to say or do, because I was engaging with my own feelings of loss.

The real issue in the need for compassion from others is the complexity of Opportunity Costs, discussed under "O". My children lost their father to cancer. Having a disabled mother just kept them in the medical loop of death, disease, and disability. I don't know many mothers or fathers who would choose that sort of childhood for their loved ones. Now you must not only deal with the frustration of your disease but also the implicit impact it has on your family.

When I am riding in a wheelchair, as I must do for long distances and trips, I am often ignored or rushed by, like a giant bug clogging up the sidewalk. This is something that doesn't happen every outing, but it happens enough that I don't enjoy going out. Sitting and seeing – not people's faces, but their butts or crotches just becomes tedious. I am unable to turn my head so looking up or down or sideways is not an option. I feel trapped.

When I am feeling jaded and dejected, I am reminded of how often people will go out of their way to help. This will be discussed under kindness, because once you get out of your comfortable routine, you realize how tricky and fast-paced the modern world is, it is just not accommodating to slow-mo people. When I find a tolerant and helpful person, I have been so humbled and grateful that kindness and solicitude have not completely evaporated from modern life.

But quite sadly, I often get a different reception. Being rarely acknowledged gets old, like you are no longer a significant player in the game of life. Because now that I am old, there is an expected dismissal of my presence or my importance.

COURAGE

As a child in the 50's, there was no one more powerful or courageous than Superman. Such are the things of fantasy – a man who could jump tall buildings, etc. etc. Then, in the 90's, we had a different Superman, a beautiful man named Christopher Reeve. He fell from a horse and severed his spine. He became a paraplegic in a matter of minutes. His steely resolve to recover was raw courage on display.

After an 8-year struggle, he sadly succumbed to his injuries. No longer the fantasy man, but the real and very vulnerable human being. Courage comes in so many unexpected places.

From my point of view, athletes and military people are the best equipped to face these cataclysmic challenges. Athletes and military people know how to train, how to reach goals, how to compete and challenge their bodies. Not sure if the mantra "No pain, no gain" is as popular as it used to be, because we are realizing there are limits to endurance and strength training.

I am not talking about the Olympics or battle readiness, I am talking about getting out of bed and trying to exercise a body that, in no way, wants to move. Your body will resist your efforts. Your pain will tell you it isn't worth it, but your mind will know there is a pay-off if you can only muster the courage to challenge your pain. Remember the old adage, "A coward dies a thousand deaths, a hero dies but one."

D

DEPRESSION

Inevitably, when I fill out forms at a new doctor's office, there is a section inquiring, regardless of the specialist, "Are you depressed? Have you lost the joy of living?" That kind of question.

For me, it is insidious. Of course, we all get down from time to time. Being immobile and in pain does not make for happiness. So, I wonder at this line of questioning. I know there are personality disorders that displace their angst and manifest physical symptoms, but I want to take a poll. If you were just diagnosed with a life-altering disease that comes with pain and disability, would you feel depressed and joyless?

I get why they are asking this question, to ascertain if there is a hidden mental illness inside you that is manifesting in physical symptoms. I was 29 years old when I got this disease. It is genetic. My aunt was in a wheelchair by the time she was 40. I am not a psycho nut case that just wants attention, and trust me I have been treated as such many times over the years. The back doctors who told me "to live with it", the weight doctors who told me "just push away from the table", the joint specialists who told me, "you're too young."

This is why I go to therapy, because these are harsh realities to embrace but there will never be help in a medical doctor's office. I am wondering if I broke down, sobbed, and was sad whether they would insist I go to a mental hospital instead of an orthopedic hospital. I am wondering what would happen if I answered, "Yes, I am depressed." Would they find me a therapist? I find getting the right therapist is essential and I highly recommend it because disability is a disrupter and you're going to need help with your new reality. But therapists are expensive, and quite honestly, there are good ones and bad ones, just like car mechanics. Find the right one for you.

Mental health is a subject near and dear to me, because I have had several members of my family riddled with personality disorders, addiction, or mood disorders. I, myself, have a Masters Degree in Clinical Psychology because I wanted to understand the motivation and ideation of those family members.

I have had therapy on and off for the 47 years I have had this disease, but NOT ONE of my surgical problems had its genesis in my mind. My mind and mental health are what have enabled me to survive 17 surgeries and 47 years of a challenging and painful disease.

So often, women who were not compliant or difficult were institutionalized, with no recognition or tolerance that maybe something might be wrong at home, like abuse or domestic violence. I mention this, because now on these same doctor's forms, they will ask, "Do you feel safe?"

And I want to scream, "Nobody is safe – have you seen the way of the world? Fires, wars, insane politicians." But, of course, that would be greeted as a sign of my instability, not a call to arms to change the world. I have been working on that my whole life, and now I realize, I can only change myself.

The overlap between physical and mental illness is real and needs to be explored. I am not sure asking patients on a form if they are depressed is a clinical approach to this solution, but I imagine it is a start.

We really don't understand humans, do we? How many humans even know their own body? How many teeth do we have? How many vertebrae? How many joints? How many anatomical systems? AI tells me we have 16 anatomical systems. Who knew? You can look them up if you have a mind to, the point is, we really don't know our bodies well at all.

Not only that, but how many humans know their own mind? There is a buzz of a storm in most mentally challenged people. A basic tenet of mental health is to know thyself, and that can often take a lifetime.

DIET

In 2005, I had a wonderful family doctor who told me glutens were inflammatory for arthritis and she recommended I remove them from my diet, which I did. Immediately, I felt the relief in my body and I was able to shed some unwanted pounds. Little did I know what a maelstrom being gluten-free would incite.

In those days, there were no gluten-free products. I thought it was mainly bread and pasta. Little did I know how vast the world of glutens truly is. Add to that, I am lactose-intolerant. Makes me unpopular at parties and restaurants, unless the host is kind and has similar problems, or the chef is adaptable.

Nowadays, there are endless opportunities to eat gluten-free, but it is still not fully embraced by the general public, in fact there is a heap of scorn from some populations with the implicit message: just get along. "You gotta go along to get along," but the whole thing is there is no way "to get along" when you are immobilized.

Closely related to diet is digestion. It is awful to lie in bed and to have a disgruntled stomach. There is gas and cramping and diarrhea and constipation and vomiting. A whole host of complexities come from your stomach, which has been labeled "the second brain". For me, my stomach was the whistleblower of my disease which presented with projectile vomiting.

Add to this, the complexities of drug regimens, rarely accepted by the stomach without a measure of protest. Take with food, don't take with food, take at night, take in the morning, take when necessary, take when you are sitting up, take when you are lying down. Boggles the mind, really.

For me, drug therapy was not successful. I was prescribed a medicine in 2005 which I cannot name because Big Pharma would swat me down like a pesky flea. But this drug, which is advertised on television today, blurred my vision. In the advertisement on TV, they file a disclaimer: "May cause blurred vision." Oh Lord, did it ever. I couldn't read a regular book for almost twenty years but early days, thanks to my techie granddaughter, we figured out how to use an e-book which worked for a while, but then it didn't.

I finally had four eye surgeries, and my vision is semi-restored. But I am 76 years old now, and I would have really loved those 20 years back. That's the problem, isn't it? You don't get a do-over. There's no going back to days when reading was my primary joy.

DOCTORS

Doctors come in all shapes, sizes, and categories. Not all are created equal, just like the rest of us. There are alternative doctors, which include chiropractors, acupuncturists, hypnotherapists, and a host of other healers. There are medical doctors who are divided into two categories – medical doctors which include primary care, cardiology, neurology, gastroenterology, nephrology, to name just a few. The other category is surgeons – the ones who can cut you open and fix the inside parts. People get confused about these separations. There are even more categories, doctors of osteopathy, doctors of dentistry. So, when someone says, "My doctor recommends," I wonder what doctor they are talking about.

Early days in my disease, I found chiropractors could adjust my neck and straighten my spine which provided great relief. My father almost disowned me, because it was the 1970s and Alternative Medicine was not seen in a friendly light.

For twenty-five years, I used any form of Alternative Medicine I could. After nothing helped, my friendly chiropractor looked at me one day and said, "It's time for you to see a surgeon. Eastern medicine has done all it can, and now you need Western Medicine." And Western Medicine delivered.

E

ENERGY

When your life becomes interrupted by whatever force disabled you, you will, if like me, become understandably despondent. How am I going to get my life back?

In the early 2000s, I was seeing a remarkable rheumatologist. While I was waiting in the waiting room, I picked up a copy of Arthritis Today – a magazine I didn't even know existed.

The article I read was focused on the sense of exhaustion one gets from arthritis which takes your energy and vitality in unexplainable ways. I was in my 50s then, so I arrogantly poo-pooed it. The writer of this article might be overwhelmed and exhausted, but not me. I was going to do everything I could to keep my energy up. After all, I had two teenagers at home. I needed my wits and my energy.

Of course, now, 20 years later, I get exactly what that article was trying to communicate. Your energy will be one of the first things to go, along with mobility.

My pain doctor used to tell me to do "ONE THING A DAY" so I could feel human and not a worthless, bed-ridden invalid. I love the word INVALID, the definition is "a person made weak or disabled by illness or injury." But to me, it sounded like I was in-valid – no longer a player in the game of life.

ENVIRONMENT

I already mentioned my bedroom. I am a cheerful, light-hearted person when I am not riddled with pain. Therefore, I want my home to reflect that energy, not a dark and depressive place. I feel so much gratitude that I have had the resources to stay in my own home, to be the captain of my own ship, and not subject to someone else's rules.

Joint replacement surgeries are complicated. When I had my first knee replaced in 2003, knee replacements weren't as common as nowadays and usually required a minimum of 5 days in the hospital. When I am hospitalized after surgery, I like to keep the environment in my room peaceful despite so much pain. I play the music meditation channel. I do not need action when I am healing, I need peace and contemplation. Music transports me like no other medium. I find comfort there. Because I do understand that diverting your brain from pain takes distraction, try to create whatever environment makes you happy. If you are an avid sports fan, then put up a poster or watch ESPN non-stop. At this stage of the game, we all get to create our own nest, our own comfort station.

I have never gone to a rehab facility after my surgeries. I

was lucky enough to go home, which I realized placed a burden on my family. I hate being a burden. I like being the provider for my family, not the WEAK LINK for them to wait on during my convalescence and rehabilitation from surgery. But in the early days in my surgeries, I didn't know about rehab centers. Somehow, we got through it, and I am forever grateful for their loving care.

EXERCISE

Now we have come to my favorite topic. As I mentioned, I was an active kind of kid. As a child, I was the only girl amongst a sea of boys which included my two older brothers, so I learned to play like a boy. That means you are fearless and tough, because girls were seen as sissies and if you acted like a sissy, you were OFF THE FIELD.

As I was fearless and tough, I was accepted in their games. That conditioning has been immeasurably valuable to me as I faced the adversary that is Arthur the abuser.

There are really two motivations to exercise – to help your body and to ease your mind. I embrace both. My body wants strength conditioning, my mind knows I must stretch and nurture my limbs to remember I am capable of moving, just not like I did before.

As mentioned, I was competitive. In swimming, I was asked

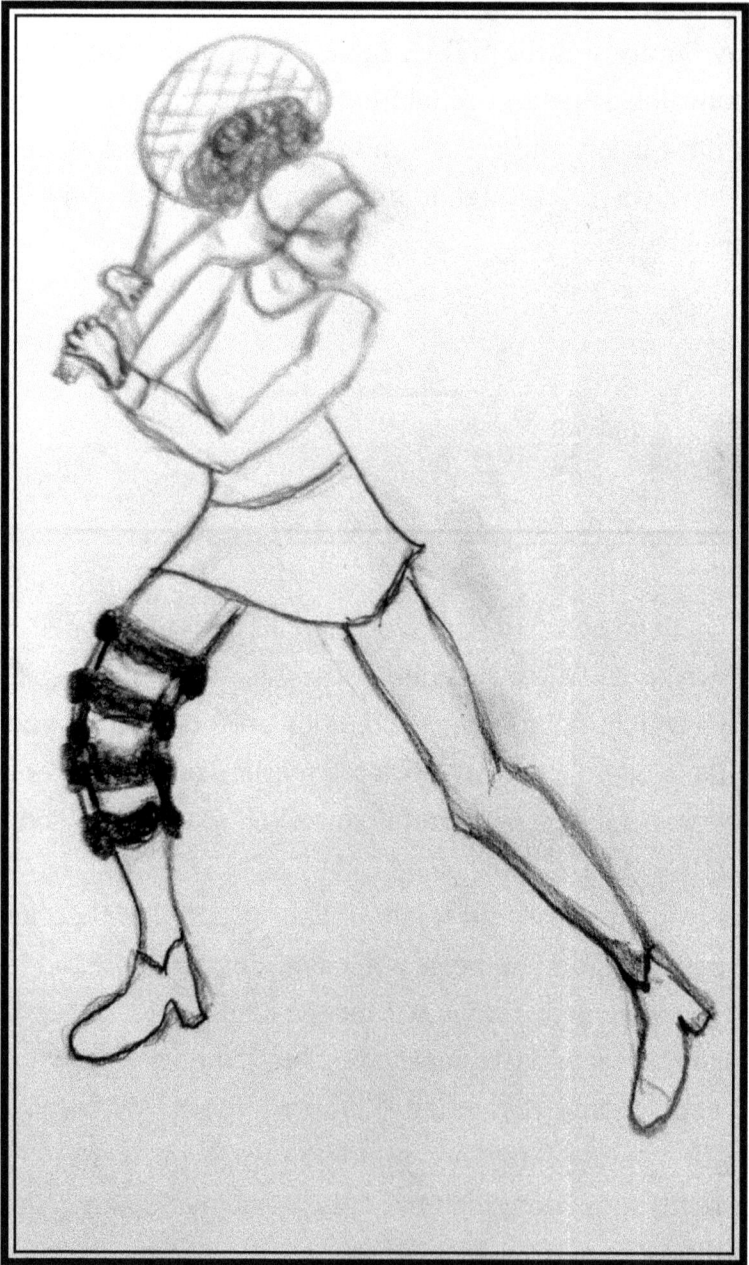

to train for the Olympics, not a choice for me because the swim club was in a different state, and I did not have a family who would champion my success. In tennis, I was an A- player. My inability to move fluidly was more obvious on land than in the water.

And my favorite activity was horseback riding, which triggers a lot of reactions. Mainly, that it is an aristocratic discipline – only for the rich and famous. But for me, it was a scrappy space. I was 11 years old when I bought my first horse for $50, and trust me, in 1959, that was not enough to buy a quality horse. It was the money I earned from babysitting and collecting empty soda bottles to redeem at the store. I still marvel that I could babysit at eleven years of age and get paid for it. But times were different then, and maybe we trusted children more than we do now. Not sure but I am sure that babysitting job, which I held until I left for college, allowed me to have the love of my life at that time, my horse.

It was the late 1950s and many of my friends at school also had horses. I grew up in the West where there were still wide-open spaces. We would meet after school to go riding, we would have horse shows on the weekend and have club meetings. Our high school had a Billy Bob Rodeo Club and I became a barrel racer. For a kid who never wanted to go home, it was my sacred, safe place. But horses can be dangerous if you don't know what you're doing, and believe me, at 11 years old, I didn't have a clue. I learned over the years, but the lesson came with a lot of falling off. This, relaxing when you are falling, has been a skill set I had no idea would become so valuable to me and which I will try to describe under FALLING.

I have listed the exercise my mind and spirit wanted, but sadly, back then, doing preparation for your body for your sport was not common practice. You just got out there and DID IT! It was not emphasized at the time that strength training truly begins in a gym. Lifting weights, working on cardio, stretching, and challenging the right muscle groups – these are, sadly, skills I learned later in life. A bit too much later. The damage was already done. Not that anything could have mitigated my disease as I was extremely fit when it hit. Fitness would be the key to my later success in rehabbing from surgeries.

F

FALLING

My descent from a horse's back was my training to hit the ground and not get hurt. Sometimes, being hurt was inevitable – being dragged, getting stepped on, and gathering new scars. None of that rough and tumble danger ever deterred me or frightened me. Fearless, and a bit foolish, I carried on.

I do understand 95 percent of people reading this book have never had the occasion to ride a horse, much less fall off one. So, let's address the fear of falling. A concern of the utmost importance. Last week three of the seniors in our community had horrific falls. It can happen to anyone in a blink of an eye.

The critical issue is to relax. If you brace and tense up in flight, you will crack something. Think of it this way: a hard surface, like an eggshell, will crack like Humpty Dumpty, who was lucky he didn't crack open. But if you make yourself soft and pliable, the fall will not be as catastrophic.

Of course, the idea is not to fall at all. But these things are not predictable, so we are often surprised when we trip or stumble or go flying through the air. The fall might not hurt you, but you cannot get up. I am in this category. I have not been able to get myself up off the ground for over 20 years. Providence has been watching over me, because I haven't had a fall where I couldn't crawl to a chair or some support to hoist myself up.

I don't watch cable television, but I do get the scent of the scorn out there for people like me. I've heard comedians joke about someone looking as if they are a candidate for those commercials. I have seen enough print commercials to realize how pathetically my people are portrayed. Nice to make fun of people struggling, eh? The sport of the able-bodied making a joke out of old and disabled people saddens me, but mostly it makes me angry and reminds me the world isn't a safe haven for those of us who can't get off the floor if we fall. Guess I just can't take a joke.

Nowadays, I wear a watch. It senses if I fall or am in distress. Sometimes it is over-sensitive and asks me if I have fallen when I have not, but this apparatus gives me a secure feeling. My daughter or a friend can come hoist me off the floor, or my phone can call 911 and get me help. Fortunately, in the 18 months I've worn it, I have not needed it. I really love the freedom of living alone and do not want to lose that privilege, so I travel cautiously and slowly around my house, as I do when I go out. Rushing or hurrying is an invitation to a fall, and we don't want that, ever.

FOMO

Fear Of Missing Out. I don't know when this became a popular phrase, but I first had it explained to me about six months ago. Disabled people got used to this many, many moons ago. Because for us, it is the Reality Of Missing Out or ROMO.

If you are a person who is trying to hold down a job or a family or a life, you will be challenged more than an elderly person who is getting ready to retire. I must speak from the perspective of arthritis, because that is the form of disability I have. It is considered an affliction of the elderly, 70% of the people with arthritis are over 65.

As someone who was only 29 when I got diagnosed with this condition, I was treated with suspicion. I was not OLD enough to have problems, even though the x-rays and tests showed my degeneration. Therefore, I was often considered as a whining malingerer, not someone who really needed help.

Before my spinal fusions, I had seen at least 3 doctors who offered no solution – just walk more or bed rest, it was one of the two.

I read a statistic that Arthritis is responsible for $100 billion in lost revenue due to illness and pain.

My confusion is that the 30% of people who are under 65 that have this disease are causing that much impact on our economy? Because the elderly are expected to retire anyway, right? So, 20 million people missing work seems to be the most pressing issue?

For me, these are 20 million people who are missing their children's lives, missing fun, missing love, missing music, missing sports, missing friends, missing jogging, missing bike riding, missing skiing, missing walking the dog, missing sitting in a park, missing fishing, missing concerts, missing recitals, missing weddings, missing funerals, missing volcanoes, missing oceans, missing yoga, missing church, missing charity events – the beat goes on and on with all the FOMOs which turn into ROMOs.

Seriously, there is more to this than Missing Out. These are lives permanently changed. If you are someone reading this book and you are one of them, or someone who loves or lives with them, or someone who cares for or about them: Thank you. Thank you for taking a moment to understand this confusing, complicated, and challenging condition.

———————

FRUSTRATION

This feeling is ever present every day. The myriad of tasks I can no longer perform that my Able-Bodied former self could, like driving a car or getting around without the cumbersome complications of my crippled carcass. I try to accept these feelings as frustration and not resentment.

If you get locked into LIFE ISN'T FAIR and want to bang on about it for years and years and years, go ahead, but I am not too sure you will be rewarded with the audience you expect. Because endless annoyance is not a good healing place.

When I am in a frustrating situation, I try to remember we are all doing our best. Few people can put themselves in the shoes of a disabled person because it is a big leap for some.

I remember when I was in Graduate School studying for a

Masters in Psychology. One of our professors took the class to a supermarket. She had brought glasses with glass lenses, but no correction and she had us rub Vaseline on the lenses, she wanted us to see what blurred vision does to our sense of safety. We were to put plugs in our ears to reduce our ability to hear. Some of us were to use canes, some walkers, and some grocery carts. She commissioned us to fulfill a grocery list and meet at the front of the store when we were finished.

Many people bitched and groaned how utterly stupid this was. But for me I understood because I had an elderly father. Now that I have lost the clarity of my vision, the steadiness of my walking gait, and the comfort of being in commercial spaces, it has been driven home and helps me accept my overall frustration with shopping for anything.

G

GARDENING AND COOKING

There is tremendous pleasure one can get from tending living, growing things, or making edible delights in the kitchen. Of course, there are some who are shuddering at the suggestion. You want me to do what?

Even if it is a house plant on your windowsill, there is a little life in your world. I've always been in love with gardening and have had a variety of gardens and flower beds, plus my house is generally festooned with plants. For me, they bring hope and excitement for the future. But some of you don't have that background or confidence, I hope you can change your mindset.

Often I hear the same disclaimer when someone who can't boil an egg says, "I can't cook." For gardeners, I hear the defense, "I have a brown thumb. I kill everything I touch." Both of these disciplines, cooking and gardening, are a process of trial and error. Many people are so afraid of failure, they stop trying.

The reality is we can all grow things if we try. We can learn not to over-water, the right amount of light, and the optimal pots and soil. It can be something you learn, and it can open a whole new window in your world. It is something you have time for which you probably didn't before.

The added benefit of gardening is it will take you outside in a sedate fashion. SLOW MO gardening is the idea. Nothing grows in a rush, so take your time, get dirty, get hot, get wet – at least you're getting out. Also, once you plant something, it is fun to anticipate it popping up through the soil. It is a life force as old as time.

For me, the early days of my recovery precluded gardening or cooking. For both of these activities, one needs to stand up or be mobile. Hard to cook from a wheelchair, although I am sure it could be adaptable. The point is, try to fix your own nutritious food. Your body will feel gratitude. There are services that deliver food to your door. Takeout comes to your door, but if you are picky like me, I prefer to make my food at home.

Please try to expand yourself either in the garden or on the apartment windowsill or in the kitchen, because the more you embrace the riches of life – good food and good atmosphere, the happier and healthier life becomes.

GRIEF

Grief and pain are the major obstacles to healing. Grief is the unimaginable loss being recycled over and over in your beleaguered mind. You've lost something you can never get back – a sense of innocence of a time gone by. Whether it is someone dear you lost, or it is the loss of your physicality, it is a dark and pressing feeling of being lost in a void.

Elisabeth Kubler-Ross wrote about the denial of death and the navigation of grief back in 1969. Brilliantly, she mapped out five stages of grief or loss. They are: Denial, Anger, Bargaining, Depression, and Acceptance. For me personally, and professionally, the rationale behind her research coincided with my own development as a human being.

Having lost my mother when I was eight, no one explained the pain to me. My father was a very stoic man of Native American ancestry. He stoically learned to stuff his feelings to survive. But if you are in a personal battle with an aggressive disease, as I was, I think it is important to acknowledge the role grief and eventual acceptance play in your journey. No one can understand your ordeal because it is specific to you, and it is wise to try to dig down and figure out what's happening. Some people are locked in a state of perpetual rage.

Unresolved grief is rough because our society wants nothing to do with grief. We want people engaged, bubbly, enterprising, and entertaining with no obvious problems. There is nothing entertaining about grief, unless television or a blockbuster movie portrays someone else's grief.

Grief is very specific to each person but has a universal and global understanding. War torn zones, cancer wards, pain clinics – these are spaces rife with grief. Think of the Wailing Wall. I believe there is no way to CHEER THINGS UP. One must ride the waves of loss and despair. It is important. If you stuff the grief into the inner recesses of your heart and don't shake it out, it will haunt you until your end of days. Grief counselors are extraordinarily helpful here, and there are YouTube channels that can help if a therapist is too expensive.

GUILT

This is an emotion that travels with grief. I ALWAYS felt guilty my girls had to care for me and didn't have a carefree childhood. I felt guilty I could not lift my grandchildren but had to have them placed in my lap for cuddling and burping. Most of us do not want to burden our families, or burden our friends, and we embrace the reality that our existence does create extra work for the ones we love.

This is a two-way street. I had the privilege of caring for loved ones who were suffering – cancer with my mom who died when I was 8. AIDS felled a beloved brother who had contracted it from a blood transfusion in 1983. Trust me when I tell you that AIDS is extraordinarily painful. And the last was my father, who had Alzheimer's and ended up in a care facility for 4 years. The mental confusion that comes with Alzheimer's is so heartbreaking. My father had been a very successful executive. A man with an amazing intelligence regressed to being infantile.

For all of those loved ones, I felt guilty I couldn't save them, and the grief I felt was almost unbearable. I think grief and guilt are very human and common emotions. The trick is not to let them run your life.

H

HEALTH

Being healthy is a state of mind and a product of your genetics, behavior, and choices. I may have a vicious disease, but I try to treat the rest of me with as much love and care as I can.

Eating healthy, for me, was the first building block in my road to health and started in 1978 after I had been hospitalized, because I knew I had a rough disease but had no idea at the time what a game changer that disease would become. My mom had died when I was 8, and I had a beautiful daughter who had just turned that age. I started reading about healthy living – eating organic, limiting calories, getting exercise, and being around positive people.

I am now 76 and I am convinced as I now live in a retirement community, I made the right choice. At my age, you can tell the ones in my age group who worked at fitness and health. I callously think the other, unhealthy ones, were stubborn and wanted to eat whatever they wanted and to do whatever suited their fancy. I realize that has a heavy load of judgment attached to my attitude, but people who don't treat themselves well become draining. I would say weight and mobility are the common complaints.

For me, I was a mother, and the choices I made were because I loved being a mother, and didn't want to be responsible for my own ill-health because of selfish choices. I had enough to deal with dysfunctional Arthur eating all my cartilage.

Processed foods, to me, are the nemesis of the American diet. Quick, fast food is truly the enemy of your body. It might soothe your soul, but I am thinking a healthy body has a better spiritual home because there isn't the angst that bad food brings.

As I see the seniors who lumber around the pool carrying 50 or more pounds of excess weight, I want to cry. What are you doing? Your body is really struggling with that poundage. Weight is a topic all its own and will be addressed under W, because it is one of the central challenges for many people's road to health.

There is more to health than diet and exercise, there is mindset or attitude. I used to tell my children that "Attitude is Everything."

I think this emphasis on mindset was established by my father. He rarely had time to read to me, so when he did, I think I remembered every word of every story. The one he particularly liked to read to me was "The Little Engine That Could." The mantra of the little engine that saved the whole circus was, "I can, I can, I think I can."

What is your attitude toward a healthy lifestyle? If you think it is something only for the rich and famous, you're sunk already. We all have the means and the right to be healthy. As far as means go, I get that nutritious food and fancy yoga classes might be out of some people's reach, but vegetables are one of the cheapest foods out there, and all of us can get a good stretch in, even if bedridden, because there are so many coaches out there shouting WELLNESS – please open your ears and hearts to them.

HOSPITALS

I would like to say hospitals run with efficiency, safety, and perfection – unfortunately, I cannot. They are run by humans, and humans are as humans do, they are imperfect. The modern mission is to have NO MISTAKES – EVER!! That is the mission, but remember it is run by humans. Shit happens, mistakes occur.

One just prays it is not your time – there is a great leap of faith one must have to even enter the place. Trust me, most people would prefer to be somewhere else. But your body has malfunctioned on some level, and you need help. Other than having a baby, the hospital is to humans what an automobile repair shop is to your car. You are just going to take longer to recover than a broken auto part.

I have had seventeen surgeries, and only four of them were outpatient procedures. When I get to the hospital, I know whether I will be going home afterwards or not. When I get to the hospital, I start praying. "Please let me wake up to my children. Please do your jobs well. Please let me live. Please let me be mobile." These are my thoughts and prayers prior to surgery. Please let the doctor feel well – hope he had a good breakfast, no fights with the wife, that sort of thing. There are so very many variables that can go wrong. We all know when they do. We just have to pray that they won't.

From 1975 to1983, I worked in a hospital and knew how it was run. It was a Catholic hospital where the nuns were the main nursing force, and they still wore their habits. Administering mercy and medicine were equally important.

Sadly, in 1983, hospitals were no longer non-profit, and they could operate as a business. This was a devastating change, in my mind, for the future of modern medicine. Big Pharma and the insurance companies are now driving the bus, and like all businesses, their primary objective is profit, profit, profit.

HYDRATION

There are fluids you need to put into your body and fluids that are already in your body. These are really critical elements. The primary fluid we need to ingest is water. If you have a heavy drug regimen, water will help push the meds to their desired target. If you are fighting with your stomach and have indigestion, then water can be your friend.

Another sad evolution when health was the intention, because people started carrying plastic water bottles with disastrous effects on the environment. Yes, we all need to drink more water, especially seniors, but plastic bottles are the worst because the water gets warm and the bottles get weak. Personal thermos bottles can be quite the fashion statement in some areas.

However, I live in a retro-retirement community and I always carry my own water bottle. I have been asked, "What's in that bottle? Tequila?" This is at a 10 o'clock water exercise class. Are you so unaware of your bodies' need for fluid and the unintended environmental impact of plastic, that your hydration and your own health are compromised?

Fluids in your system are just as critical and more incomprehensible because there are so many choices out there: juices, sodas, energy drinks, alcohol, milk, and good old water. Juices and sodas can be tricky because they often have added sugar, and too much sugar risks diabetes.

Alcohol was my go-to pain reliever for many years. I once told a doctor this, and she immediately labeled me an alcoholic. Pity that. The moderate use of alcohol can relieve stress in ways many other things can't. Remember those cavemen? I am sure there were some fermented fruits or potatoes that helped take the edge off. Taking the edge off is all you can really hope for when in high levels of pain.

I take a prescriptive medication for my arthritis that can be rough on the liver and kidneys. I get my blood drawn once a month to keep tabs if things get out of kelter. The key to my success with those blood tests is to drink LOTS of water. Which means lots of trips to the toilet. If you are able-bodied, this can be inconvenient and annoying, but if you are disabled, it limits your desire to be out in public. Public toilets are not reliably friendly to disabled people.

So remember – water, water, water!

IMAGINATION

Imagination has been my best companion and has kept me positive and light during very dark and painful times, like when I was bedridden for about 10 years. Not to mention the painful reality of before and after surgeries, I wanted to escape. Fortunately, I was gifted with a great imagination. I can lie in bed and pretend I am riding a flying horse that can take me to all the places I would love to see, or places where I remember being very happy, or I can have a long visit with someone I have loved and lost. I can pretend I am dancing, swimming, riding a bike, and being outdoors. Because imagination can help you escape the world of an invalid's reality, which is truly grim.

Sadly, children are not encouraged to imagine in school. They must learn all their 3 R's and Creativity is not an R, neither is Art or Music, and neither, honestly, is arithmetic. What a loss to think these things have been suppressed for the almighty world of Math and Science. We will need a new Oppenheimer to undo what the other one has wrought. Time is of the essence in the space and weapons of war race. God forbid we fall behind.

But to me, the beauty of mankind is the capacity for creation and beauty. Keats wrote about truth and beauty. Also, think of the axioms, The truth shall set you free, and beauty is in the eye of the beholder, etc. etc.

———————

INJECTIONS

Some of us have a fear of needles. I, too, remember those childhood shots that hurt like hell and terrified me. But we must grow up quickly if we have a health challenge. Injections are not only a preventative tool, like flu shots, but they are also a treatment tool. Besides alleviating pain, like steroidal injections, they can also give a surgeon a blueprint of your pain to discover if they are on the right path to ameliorate your pain. Injections tell the medical people if they are in the right area for your treatment.

If recollection serves me well, I believe my love affair with pain-relieving injections began with my knees. I would get Synvisc injections, which are a gel-like mixture that lubricates the knees and have an expiration date of six months. I did this for years, then they just stopped working. Time for some surgical intervention.

At first, my surgeon wanted to do an osteotomy, "a procedure for cutting and reshaping a bone to treat problems at a joint." The problem was, when the doctor opened me up, my bone was so deteriorated, he had nothing to work with, and he closed me back up. I spent the night in the hospital, which was a bit scary for my family. The September 11th attacks had just happened.

Everyone was edgy and jumpy, me included. I was upset I had gone through this for nothing. Didn't the MRI and CT scan show the degeneration in my leg? The problem was, I was just 53 years old, much too young to warrant a knee replacement.

So finally, this reluctant surgeon knew I needed my left knee replaced. Once that was over, and a rough surgery that is, my friends, my hip started causing me pain. Again, too young to have this level of arthritis, so my surgeon wanted to do a diagnostic injection. The plan was to inject my left hip with cortisone. If I could walk without pain, then BINGO – we've got the culprit.

This was done in his office. I laid on an x-ray table, and this nice, gentle, jolly man who had operated on me three times before, stuck a needle the length of a conductor's baton into my hip. To this day, I think that was one of the more painful events of my long, painful journey. It burned with incredible intensity. I looked at him with tears in my eyes and realized I had been asleep when he had done more painful things to me. It stilled me. The power of pain to completely immobilize a person was never more evident than in that moment. It was also the magical moment when I realized I was Humpty Dumpty – could all the King's men put me back together again?

I realize that hip injection is the extreme and would probably be done in a surgical center nowadays. Since that day, I have never been confronted with such a high level of pain with injections.

Before my back fusion, I needed three or four epidural injections for my doctor to understand the extent of my degeneration. I wanted to include this, because we assume doctors are omniscient and can see into our wounds, but the reality is, they need a roadmap, and injections give them the particulars of the scene that is your body. They don't want any surprises or wrong turns.

Please don't alarm yourself by this gruesome story, because so many of the injections I get are for relief. The routine ones I have had are steroidal trigger point injections. I have had those in my foot, my jaw, my knees, my hips, my shoulders, my neck, and my back. I love them. But, again, they have a shelf life of 3 months. This is highly frustrating. If you can give me relief for 3 months, why can't it be more permanent? A question for another time, I fear.

ISOLATION

We have all just experienced different levels of isolation with the Covid pandemic. For the first time in my memory, people were presented with being confined. Having already been labeled a "shut in", it wasn't too dramatic because I rarely left home anyway. Sadly, some folks were climbing the walls. I am wondering if they were isolated in solitary, or isolated with a family. The sad news about domestic abuse is its prevalence –1 in 3 households report problems. And those are only the households who report in. Disabled people are targets for the cruelty of domestic abuse.

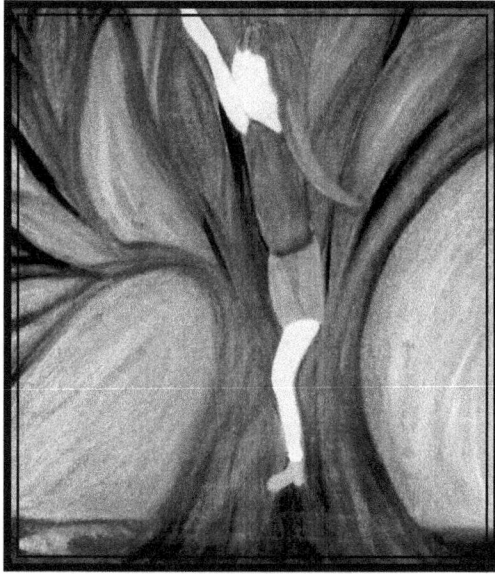

The American Psychological Association reports that women with disabilities have a 40% greater chance of intimate partner violence than women without disabilities. I can only imagine what door Covid isolation opened to that nightmare.

For me, the presence of my daughter made all the madness bearable. However, she was working and traveling some, so not always home. We must learn to self-nurture, to be self-reliant.

For me, seeing other people was mitigated by my being connected to friends and family via the phone, which is my usual way of connection. I haven't driven a car in 12 years and I haven't been able to go on walks by myself for many years. Remember when employees were working from home? We could hear the children in the background, but who cared? We got connected.

For me, the pandemic was same old, same old in many ways. I think some people got antsy and panicked. For me, I started

Papier Mache to pass the time away and to use up those annoying Wednesday newspaper sales ads. I got sick of just throwing them in the recycling so I watched YouTube channels and learned to Papier Mache. Besides the newspaper, all you need is flour and water.

We had four old wooden tables my daughter's ex-roommate had given her. I decided to beautify them. I had a lifelong love of mosaics and had never had the time to learn the skill. YouTube had a tutorial and Amazon helped so much when I needed supplies to make the mosaic tables.

Also, I could order gardening supplies, and art supplies. I talked endlessly on the phone to the people I love who are usually too busy to have much gab time. I managed the isolation because I was very accustomed to it.

My experience with isolation came at a very young age. My mother was dying of cancer, and I was eight-years-old and missed the age cut-off for summer camp like my brothers. I was the only child left at home. I was not allowed in the house once my father left for work, because we had a housekeeper named Bessie. Bessie didn't like children, so she shushed me out of the house whenever she could. Fortunately, it was summer, so I didn't freeze or anything.

We had just relocated to that city, so there were no family friends and no familiar playmates to occupy me while my mother lay inside the house, suffering from a disease that had required surgery after surgery and was eating her alive.

I spent most of my time playing with my dogs and sitting in a tree by the side of the road waiting for my father to come home. Waiting for my mother to die. I realized as I got older that Bessie was trying to keep the house quiet for my mom. The year was 1957 and television did not have 24-hour programming. Things came on in the evening. I wonder how my mother endured it, but she did. And it is from her that I have gathered my courage through my life. She didn't complain.

I believe it is because I spent a summer sitting in a tree waiting for my mother to die, that I learned how to handle pain and isolation. I knew there was a God or Universal energy, and I prayed to that Spirit to ease my mother's end. To let her die in peace, not agony. I have always prayed for that for the people I love, and I believe those prayers are answered. Despite our resistance, death will come to us all one day. It is part of the human equation.

Modern technology has obviated isolation. The privacy I knew and grew up with is a thing of the past. I get texts, emails, ads, scams, pleas for money – you all know the drill. We are under the same siege. But it isn't the adults I am so concerned about, it is the children.

Modern day parents seem to shove a cell phone or iPad in their kids' faces to shut them up, to pacify them. Seriously, this is a giant mistake. Children need to know how to find comfort in their own company and not seek it from others, they need to learn to soothe themselves. This is a pattern set in childhood.

It was at a very young age that I learned I was a pain warrior because I listened to my own voice, that very voice that knew my mother would die and she would be okay. What if I had just blithely been given a device or television program to numb the pain? It is a life lesson we need to learn as individuals, not join the herd mentality way too young.

Distraction and diversion are considered better options than confrontation or authenticity, eventually one will learn to avoid the reality around them and sink into an alternate universe.

A screaming child in a crib or in a car seat is not an emergency. It is annoying and the screaming sucks, but it is a rite of passage we have denied the new screen-addicted generation – the gift of learning self-soothing, of facing the moment at hand, not seeking numbness and diversion which is the ground zero of addiction. Fear and numbness are options in stress, but how much healthier to face the fear and shake out the numbness.

The story of my mother dying sounds like a dramatic soap opera kind of scenario, but the reality is we are conditioned in childhood to accept uncomfortable and unfathomable situations. It is the template of how we handle stress and pain, and yes, isolation. Because for me, it was familiar territory. I had seen my mother's scars from a young age. A double mastectomy which created a gape in her chest (there were no cosmetic fixes in those days for those scars), and a hysterectomy which was unseen to me. These surgeries required a great deal of absence.

In those days, children were not allowed in the hospital. One year, special dispensation was given on Thanksgiving, my mother's favorite holiday. My father smuggled me in to see her, hiding me under his raincoat because I was the one underage. My brothers were old enough to be seen and acknowledged.

The hospital was a place that smelled really, really bad and was super scary. I didn't want my mom to be there. I think going there helped me understand her struggle and her pain. She would not die until August, and the grace she showed during her struggle has sustained me my entire life.

When you are in a hospital bed for an operation or are

recovering from surgery, it is a very lonely time. The family will come for a visit. The playoffs will entertain us and divert us, but when the lights are off and we must sleep, we wrestle with the reality we find ourselves in. If you had a childhood full of trauma, illness, or war, then I believe it will be more difficult to feel safe. But if your strategy is to distract yourself with electronic devices and 24-hour television, you really aren't doing yourself any favors, because your primary connection is to the screen, not the people in your life.

I once stayed with a dear friend who could not turn off the television. It blared 24-7 in her house. Would have driven me mad to have the incessant noise, the commercials, the negative ad campaigns. Not my style but I accept we are not all the same in our need for comfort.

J

JEALOUSY

This takes us back to the one-legged lady in the sauna. I realized one of the reasons I didn't want to talk to her was my underlying jealousy – she could swim, and I could not. I used to be a champion swimmer, so it is a loss I grieve every day. It says so much about disability and loss, doesn't it? We are jealous of those who have not had to confront this in their lives.

My disability has prevented me from going to the weddings of people I care very much about, going on trips with friends, attending any class or gathering unless the environment is hospitable, which is rarely a guarantee. It has reduced the number of activities I can enjoy. Painting is a huge release for me, however, my shoulder surgeries have prevented my ability to paint for years at a time. I have gotten back to painting, but it is very much on a limited schedule.

So, I am not jealous for the usual reasons of money, looks, or success, I am jealous I cannot do things I enjoy. I've adapted and can find pleasure, but in days gone by, I would love to go on a hike with my daughter. We tried for many years to get on the hiking trail, but it just became more and more untenable. I am jealous of those who don't have to think twice about doing their favorite activities.

Date	Procedure	Hospital
	Right Knee	
	Right Shoulder Rotator Cuff Repair	
	Right Shoulder Diagnostic	
	Left Knee Arthroscopic Debridement	Scripps Memorial
	Left Shoulder Rotator Cuff repair	Scripps Memorial
2003 – June	Left Knee – Total Replacement	Scripps Memorial
2004 – June	Left Hip – Total Replacement	Scripps Memorial
2006 – December	Right Knee – Total Replacement	Scripps Memorial
2009 – October	Right Hip – Total Replacement	St. Francis Memorial
2011 – May	Right Shoulder – Repair	Univ CA at San Francisco (UCSF)
2014 – June	Spinal Fusion (S1 – T9)	UCSF
2015 – January	Abdominal Wall Hernia Repair	UCSF
2015 - August	Abdominal Wall Hernia Repair	UCSF
2015 – December	Spinal Fusion (T9 to top of spine)	UCSF
? – May	Cervical Fusion (C1 – C6?)	UCSF
? – May	Right Shoulder Total Replacement	UCSF

JOINT REPLACEMENT

Joint replacements are the last stop on the pain train for many orthopedic patients. When your joint gets unstable, it starts screaming to your muscles and nerves, and they, in turn, cause you immobility and pain.

Sometimes a patient is experiencing bursitis, tendinitis, or a strained muscle and misjudges it to be the joint. This causes great frustration for most patients. Fix it NOW!! Doctors really need to observe your condition over time because a joint replacement is the last choice of intervention.

I was 55 when I had my first joint replaced in 2003, it was my knee. As I mentioned before, in 2001 the surgeon had tried an osteotomy, a procedure to stabilize the existing joint with metal brackets. I was so young, it wasn't thought a knee replacement was indicated. However, when he opened up my knee, he found the bone so riddled with arthritis and unstable, he closed me up again. That was when a knee replacement became my only option. It would be my first of many joint replacements, it would also be one of the hardest recoveries.

This was the beginning of my transformation. I call it my Reverse Pinocchio Effect, I was a real girl morphing into a metallic marvel. It would take from 2003-2018 for the complete transformation but it has almost been accomplished for the major joints in the body. My left shoulder is the only real joint left, although there are 350 smaller joints in your body, sort of like other celestial objects besides planets, lots of stars. It is the last major joint standing, and it will never get replaced because I am done with all that. Now that I am 76, I doubt a surgeon would even suggest it.

Joint replacements are a modern attempt to stabilize the patient so they are less pain-ridden and wobbly. As early as the 1800s there was interest in replacing parts and since then, a lot of explorations and transitions have resulted in the miracle we have today.

The first successful knee replacement in the United States was in 1968, and the hip replacement followed a year later. 1968 wasn't really that long ago when you think of the evolution of humanity.

There are significant differences in the two surgeries. The hip is a ball and socket joint. I found it to be a miraculous event. I woke up in the hospital feeling better, but the knee is a swing joint, and it is complicated. Once you get your knees replaced, you can never get down on all fours. Yoga is not going to be an option, unless you choose chair yoga which won't work if you have trouble sitting.

I am a veteran of the joint replacement world. Here is my area of expertise. When I was hospitalized in 1978 with the unremitting vomiting, it was decided I had Degenerative Disc Disease (DDD) which is specific to the neck and spine.

Later, Degenerative Joint Disease (DJD) showed up, DDD is the culprit in my neck and spine, and DJD is the culprit for my joints. So my honorariums are DDD, DJD and PSA (Psoriatic Arthritis). I wish I could list those on a CV.

Early days with joint replacements, there was a special caveat. Any dental work needed to be postponed for 2 years, and if that wasn't possible, an antibiotic regimen was required. The worry was dental decay and disease could infect the site of the joint replacement. That is now a controversial discussion, as most policies are these days. Talk to your dentist.

My knee replacements coincided with hip replacements. One weak joint can throw off the balance of the entire body. After my first knee, I had my first hip replacement. My left side was fine from a pain and mobility perspective, but what about the right side? First the knee, then the hip. The first two surgeries were done with a doctor I knew and trusted, but the second knee was done by a skilled surgeon but one without any social graces. He was rough and dismissive, and I left the city to go to better doctors. Fortunately, I found them.

After hips and knees came the spine. I had been to back doctor after back doctor until I found a remarkable surgeon who actually did something about my back. He fused it.

Last was a shoulder replacement. Shoulders are such complicated places, it is the juncture of so many muscles and mobility systems, like the neck. My shoulder replacement was a godsend because I had already had three previous rotator cuff repairs, which lasted a while, but eventually fell apart. I love my replaced shoulder and I can actually feel the titanium bar holding the works together.

This is a litany of my joint replacements. I trust yours is a shorter list and that your joint replacement surgeries go as well as mine did. Remember, you will have a ton of fun when you light up like a Christmas tree going through TSA security at airports.

JUSTICE

There is a compassionate understanding for most of us that life isn't fair. Some of us are rich and famous, some of us are poor and downtrodden, some of us are just regular folks trying to make their way. But for the disabled, it is an incessant reality, and I am afraid some of my fellow sufferers have a giant chip on their shoulders.

If we are the designated people to display the difficulties of being different, I don't understand how the general public cannot be more accommodating.

The Americans with Disabilities Act (ADA) of 1990 was a civil rights law prohibiting discrimination in employment practices and other areas of social life. I am not sure this Act was received with open arms by many institutions and businesses. We saw a proliferation of Handicapped Spaces in parking lots and ramps for wheelchairs and walkers and strollers and such. But there was also a heavy-laden resentment. So often, the handicap parking spaces were ill-placed for true and genuine access. It saddens me that profit prevails over peoples' wellbeing, but I live in a capitalist country, so I shouldn't have been surprised. Just disappointed.

K

KINDNESS

You might be wondering, what am I doing? I already listed Compassion. Compassion and Kindness are similar, but not the same. Compassion is a feeling within you. Kindness is how you act on that feeling.

I have often been overwhelmed by the kindness of strangers. It is such a lovely aspect of being human. Giving someone less fortunate a helping hand separates us from the savages, whoever they are these days? For me, it might be a limo-driven CEO who wants to bilk the common folks out of every last dime and doesn't have a social conscience AT ALL. Because business isn't about people, it is about profit, and don't forget that.

Sadly, we have an epidemic of homelessness, so if BUSINESS is the best you can do, I wonder. There are 24 hour business channels reporting profit/loss, GNP growth, jobs reports, etc. etc. There is a very profitable financial industry that prioritizes profit over humanity or environmental needs.

The contradiction to that is the airlines who are amazing at welcoming handicapped people. Even though the wheelchairs are annoying, I have never received more conscientious care. It amazes me I pay the same price as other people but get special treatment.

Now, let's talk about Big Corporations. There used to be compassionate clauses for people who have impaired sight. I have struggled for almost twenty years with diminished eyesight. Eight years ago, I was having trouble with a big-name department store over a credit card issue. I couldn't read the email and tried to call for help. For some reason, modern business thinks we should all use apps and portals and such, and if we, the customers, cannot comply, we must be penalized and spend precious moments on HOLD because some of us cannot use the portals or apps. So often, the writing on the computer is in blue which my eyes won't recognize. Time after time I am directed to talk to their AI assistant verbally or via text, when all I crave is a human. Any human. Even a grunter. Because they have no option for anyone who cannot use an app, a smartphone, or a computer.

There was a time when companies pretended to help the disabled, but that has faded. Having marginalized vision, I need a helper when it comes to computers or navigating anything to do with technology. Exceptions come to mind, like e-readers or the Stephen Hawking gizmos designed to help him communicate when ALS took his physical capacities, but not his mental ones, obviously. Very few of us have access to such an apparatus.

When I was trying to talk to the big-name department store, they directed me to a department I could reach that would help with the visually impaired and the handicapped. No one answered. I left my name and number. No one called. I just cancelled the credit card and was done with it. Guess they didn't care about my business. Not sure us elderly, disabled people are their target market, anyway.

I am still puzzled by businesses who let their customers

hang on the line for an indefinite amount of time before they get a human. They are putting machines over people, and that truly frightens me. Not sure if the machines will figure out the justice system, but I am afraid my confidence is shot. The machines already won't cooperate with the sight impaired.

The point of this is that as a disabled person, I am shut out from so much of life because of limited computer usage. We are all to become tech savvy or just resign from life. Too bad the techies aren't more kind. Too much time with machines, I'll wager.

KINESIOLOGY

This is the study of how human bodies work and move and age and grow. All that stuff a lot of us didn't recognize while it was happening. If you are a compromised person, you will need to learn this fast, because your body has just become a living laboratory.

Movement sometimes seems impossible. Trust me, I get this. All the stretching in the world won't fix a broken body part. But once that broken body part gets fixed, it is going to take some time for it to learn to work again. To move again.

Before the aftercare of Kinesiology, there is Kinesiotherapy which is preventive therapy. How you can strengthen your muscles to prevent injury. Gyms and walking paths and swimming pools and exercise classes are filled with people who got this memo. All age groups working on their bodies to be strong and flexible.

This is a critical aspect of disability, trying to minimize future damage.

Once we become injured and are recovering, Kinesiology is what will get us all back on the road again. It is a blessing and will be discussed further in Physical Therapy. Knowledge is power, so know your body and how to help it.

KISS

Keep It Simple Sweetie or Keep It Simple Stupid, if you took a business course. I prefer sweetie because I try to limit the negative speech that comes into my head. And stupid carries a lot of connotations. The counterpart to that in business, back in the day when I was working on my MBA, was KITA – Kick'em In the Ass. These days, we seem to have toned down the ass kicking, but not sure how much, as computers are really good at it.

To keep it simple, a disabled person must change their lifestyle. If you were a busy bee kind of person, you might now be a sedentary person. The word "slug" pops into my head from time to time, but I'm trying to be positive here.

The mandate for me was "to do one thing a day." Even if that one thing was brushing my teeth. But it truly is more than the simple self care tasks, it is interacting with other people. They don't really get your decrease in capacity to interact and entertain.

If you start simply with one thing – walking to the living room, going outside, sitting in a chair for a brief period of time, talking to a friend on the phone, or riding along as shot gun in a car just to get outside and shake off the cobwebs, then you can have a sense of accomplishment. Small steps lead to larger steps which lead to longer walks. Gradually, step by step, you will get stronger.

For me, I live in a seniors' community. Lots of people have get-togethers and parties. When I am invited, I must decline which often hurts the feelings of the host or hostess. These are people who don't know me well, because my mandate is: "No parties, no holiday gatherings, no music in the park, no hanging out and listening to music."

For over a year, I played Bridge at our local community center. I wondered for some time why I would feel so sick and disoriented after I played. Then my eye doctor told me fluorescent lights and ceiling fans were very toxic with my macular degeneration. I had to quit the group. I didn't want to and I have a persecution complex like, "Why do I always have to give up the things I love doing?" I thought Bridge would be a safe sort of venue for my social needs. Not so much. Also, people don't like you to quit, but if they can come to understand and accept it is not a rejection of them, it is the self-preservation of me, then I feel better.

I feel fortunate my Bridge playing friends found a way to put a table in a space with diminished light. It was a workaround, and I am grateful for their efforts. However, the chairs are a nightmare for me, so for now, I am passing on playing Bridge in a large group. Some ladies come to my house once a week, and that is social and fun. I like to keep the game light and fun.

L

LASSITUDE

Lassitude, lethargy, and limpness are often associated with laziness. Remember the slug? Well, when you have long rest and recovery times after complicated surgeries, there is an interesting dichotomy of rest versus activity. When do I rest my body? When do I challenge it?

When I had my first spinal fusion, I was told to get up and walk as much as possible. I am a Pollyanna-type patient, I do whatever is asked of me, if I can. The hallway around the ward, when circled four times, equaled one mile. Other than myself, there was another gentleman following the same mandate. Let's just say there were 24 rooms on the ward. As far as I knew, he and I were the only two marching around. Who knows if the other occupants of the ward had the same mandate to move, but I think a large percentage of people were accustomed to lassitude and might be transforming into slugs.

So many times, I have wished I were a couch potato-type of person. Someone who loved television and being waited on. I think my lassitude could last a lifetime if I had that sort of personality. But I do not, and I know there are others like me.

The essential issue is the difference between being versus becoming.

Being is the basic essence of our existence. That "what it is to be human" comment when I started this book. Being is the muscle that will keep you calm when you are unable to carry on. It is the knowledge of yourself and the world around you. It is the authentic you.

Becoming is performance. It is you as an active participant in your life. Growing up, going to school, getting the job, finding the right partner, or having a baby. That is becoming. What school are you going to? What are you going to do with your life? What do you do on your day off? How are you becoming the person you want to be?

For disabled people, we are more in the BE mode. We might make it back to becoming, like I have writing this book. Becoming can be a frustration for disabled people. What I was before, can I become again? Or must I become some new iteration of myself?

I am grateful to the surgeon who suggested I write this book. It got me out of my lassitude and prompted me into action.

LIMITATIONS

The restrictions of your disease and condition will become obvious as you progress through whatever challenge you are grappling with. The inability to put on your own socks, the accommodations of your toileting and shower needs, the restrictions in transportation and moving about, the changes in your table manners, perhaps the alteration of your speech patterns.

For me, one of the most troublesome limitations was my inability to drive a car. My cervical fusion meant I couldn't turn my head. A lot of drivers never bother to look around which leads to crash city, but for me, I couldn't even look in a rear-view mirror or the back seat. Not safe at any speed.

Luckily, these days I live in a seniors' community and drive a golf cart. I get around. But for 12 years I didn't. I was dependent on my daughters, friends, and Uber drivers. There were senior services that would provide transportation, but it was a scenario where I would have to wait with an uncertain pick-up time. One thing about people like me, we can't be in a holding pattern. We don't have WAIT time. I can't sit on a bench, can't drive my own wheelchair (much less a car), can't sit in most chairs because of my back. My limitation was the ability to go where I want, when I want. Fortunately, I have a home I love.

In this senior community, I hear people in their 80s and 90s wailing on, "What am I going to do if I can't drive?" My answer is, "Get a different sort of life." Adjust to your circumstances. Don't think rushing about and going shopping and running errands is the main mission of life. There is a greater purpose to your being. Embrace it. Keep yourself and other drivers safe by not jumping into the driver's seat. It's the cycle of life, not a punishment.

Living in a car culture means: Cars equal freedom, status, and security. Getting out of town quickly during an evacuation means I need someone to care enough about me to help me. Fortunately, I have that.

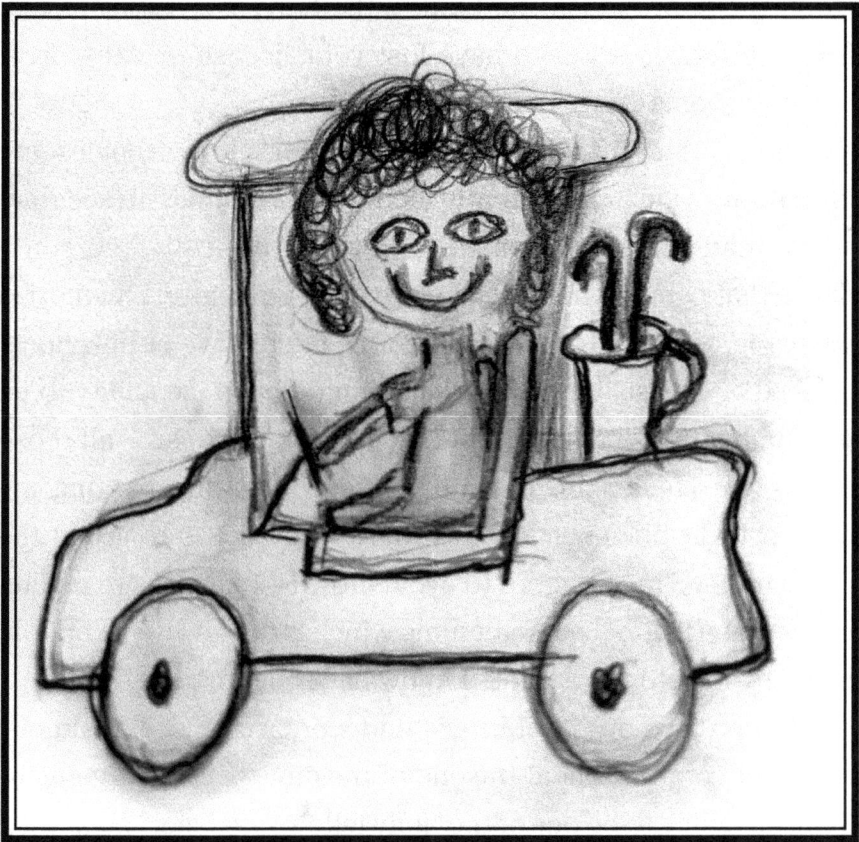

For some years, I lived in a foreign country where cars were not prolific. Very few people in large cities own cars. They simply don't need them, their feet will take them where they want to go, or they grab a bus, a subway, or a train. Where I live, however, no car means no food, no necessities of life – at least the way you were used to getting them. Nowadays, there is Amazon, there is Uber, and very often, if you're lucky, there are alternate ways of getting around. It takes some ingenuity, but it can be done. I personally love my golf cart, but I cannot drive it on some streets. Okay by me, because I can get to the grocery store, the pharmacist, the bank – the bare necessities of life. I wish those of you who have lost your license or can't drive anymore, some way to satisfy your needs.

Many other disabled people have far more troublesome limitations. One I am currently facing is the inability to see road signs, read some print on the computer, basically, the confidence that comes when one can see well. Therefore, I memorize my paths, what buttons to push on the microwave or my phone.

And of course, the most crucial limitation is the ability to be free in my body. To walk, to swim, to see well, to sit – all those events are challenging for me. Perseverance and plotting my daily path help tremendously. I know what hours to get to the pool and the grocery store to avoid crowds. I investigate restaurant seating before I go, something which is not always an option. I tend to stick to restaurants I know have comfortable seating.

We can face our limitations, find workarounds, expand our radius of comfort; but at the end of the day, we are not going to fit in, not going to be one of the "jolly fellows well met" mentality. So many times, our physical limitations are a buzzkill to us and our more able-bodied citizens.

———

LOSS

Loss is the final realization that things you cared about or things you owned or people you cared about are not coming back. Life isn't a video game or a fantasy where the fallen pop up and are back in the game. Loss is the permanent removal of something you cherished. Loss is also the alteration of your body which will never be whole again. Your life will never operate in the manner you were accustomed to because your body and mind have been altered by your entry into the world of disability.

Loss is a space where missing sunglasses, stolen treasures, failed retirement portfolios, vacation mishaps – all these sorts of losses create concern and can perhaps redirect the entire trajectory of your life. I say perhaps, because often those sunglasses, treasures, portfolios, or vacation mishaps can be ameliorated and recovered.

Recovery is impossible when a death has occurred. The loved one you lost is not coming back. Death is that final frontier we don't seem to have figured out. What happens to the people or pets we love who have passed into the great unknown? Religion helps some, but my experience with death is quite personal, and has given me a great sense of peace when it comes to dying.

The loss of a beloved pet is a rough one. These are the creatures who have lived in the world of humans and given us unconditional love. For me, my dog growing up was probably my only friend in the house. He would wag his tail and be happy to see me. That is the kind of welcome we can embrace. When we lose the life of an animal we love, we can feel quite isolated in our grief. Callous people will comment, "It's only a _____ (insert species of your pet), they aren't meant to live long lives." Pity that. I really hate losing my pets. I lost a beloved dog eighteen months ago, and I am still recovering my grief. I still miss his welcoming presence and loyal love.

Losing a loved one hurts like nothing else. It rips into your soul like a black hole. Will I ever feel joy again? Also, it challenges your faith. For me, the first loss was when I was young. A poet I cannot remember said that all present-day deaths in your life are the recreation of the first death you ever experienced.

My experience with losing loved ones began in 1957, I was eight years old when my mother died as I told you the story of the little girl in the tree. The faith I had then was that my mother would be going to a better place, a place with no pain. That faith has been rewarded because I had my own near-death experience which I have shared with many friends as they near life's end or have lost someone near and dear.

When I was about fourteen, I started getting allergy shots twice a week. In the early 1960s the protocol was to wait 20 minutes after the shot to make sure the vaccine hadn't entered the blood stream. If the vaccine entered the blood stream, anaphylactic shock would ensue constricting all your veins. This was the reason administrating doctors were also to have adrenaline also known as epinephrine at the ready in case such an event occurred.

I was young and impatient with this 20-minute ruling, I had places to go and games to play. I found a disreputable doctor who didn't make people wait. Sadly, I was to learn my lesson well, do not try to sidestep medical mandates.

It was an afternoon when my best friend drove me to get my allergy shot. We had been playing soccer and were in our shorts and tee-shirts. We walked in the office, she sat in the waiting room, and I went back to the treatment area and got my shot. As we left and got to the top of the staircase I went into full-blown anaphylactic shock. All my veins constricted turning me purple. The pain was excruciating. My poor friend was frantic. She pounded on their door. It was 5 o'clock and they had closed shop. Her frantic pounding and screaming brought the nurse to the door and she immediately sprang into action.

My good fortune was that this disreputable doctor also treated emphysema patients, so he had lots of oxygen tanks around. In anaphylactic shock, you have a matter of minutes to get oxygen to the brain, or you become a nonsensical vegetable right then. Fortunately, we got to the oxygen in time.

The other mandate of having epinephrine was ignored by this disreputable doctor, and they didn't have any. The nurse was frantically trying to get some from another office. It was the end of the day, and many of them had gone home.

Meanwhile, I was on a table and had lost all the important aspects of life – I had no vital signs. This was way before the New Age "going into the light" or "crossing to the other side" were in the public consciousness.

But I did "go into the light," there was a white tunnel with a golden haze at the end. And I heard voices, which I assumed were angels. I was floating and out of pain. I was hoping one of those voices belonged to my mother.

Meanwhile, the poor frantic nurse was shaking me and screaming, "You can't die, "you can't die," – over and over again.

I had an out-of-body experience and could see the tableau before me. I was prostrate on the table, the nurse was shaking me and screaming at me. Maybe I was worried about the nurse being blamed for my death or maybe someone had found the epinephrine and injected me just in the nick of time. Whatever force was at work, I turned around which is remarkable because I thought I heard my mother's voice in the white and golden haze. Maybe I just wasn't ready to die.

There is an amazing book that recounts the commonality with near-death experiences. It is called *Many Lives Many Masters*, which I read many years later. I was comforted to know I am not the only one who had that out-of-body experience. I have shared this story with many people nearing the end. My brother and father were comforted by my story. My father even thought he heard angels singing. If they were ever going to sing, it would have been for him. A good man has no worries about the afterlife.

Back in the doctor's room, the good news was, I survived. I was admitted to the hospital for observation. There was an enormous woman who had some sort of stomach issue who was screaming, "I am going to die. I am going to die." The nurses on the floor said, "This girl almost did die, so please be quiet and give her some peace." That quieted or calmed the woman which probably helped both of us.

Honestly, I believe many people in extreme pain wonder if they are going to die. Too bad we don't all have an "expire-by-date" so we'd know. I do believe all of us will enter the tunnel of peace where there is no pain. I have no idea what comes after the tunnel, because I turned back, but my faith tells me the spirit will live on.

MASSAGE

When I was first struck with the realization my life had changed because of a disease, I wanted to embrace all the treatment modalities I could.

First, I found a psychologist because I was struggling juggling all the demands in my life – single motherhood, small business owner, and family obligations. I was overwhelmed. I needed help both physically and psychologically. She was a godsend to me. I had a troubled childhood and didn't want to pass those treacheries onto my daughter who was seven at the time. I didn't want my disability to be her disability or limitation in life.

This psychologist recommended I see a massage therapist. This was 1978 and massage was still a shady business. All those sexual concerns of being naked and vulnerable, and then there were those yellow page ads for massages that suggested sexual complications and Happy Endings. It wasn't an easy space for me to feel comfortable in at first. But over time, I recognized the extraordinary benefit.

For 47 years, I have had weekly massage therapy treatments whenever I could. Only once did I encounter a kinky situation, but it was just a question, "Do you want a Happy Ending?" At the time, I had no idea what he meant but I declined. Later on, I realized he was talking about bringing me to orgasm. There are times in my old age I wish I could find that guy, but I am uncomfortable with strangers touching me in intimate ways, so I would probably pass.

Modern medicine is treating massage as a therapeutic modality because back in the day, it wasn't something people talked about in polite company. One of my vivid childhood memories is my mother taking me with her to a massage appointment. I had to wait in a small room while a man worked on my mother's body. I remember feeling uncomfortable and squeamish, what is that man doing to my mother?

When I mentioned I was getting massage therapy, my father was, again, in strong disagreement, and like the chiropractor, I followed my instincts and not the word of my father. Time after time, I forged my own treatment path. I am so grateful for whatever stubbornness or obstinacy kept me on my own path instead of following my father's mandates.

For me, massage has been the essence of the release of pain in my joints. Lactic acid builds up in your body, and when it is pushed around, it leaves the joint site with less swelling, and that pushing around and leaving the joint is quite a painful process, which is one reason I think people avoid massage therapy. It rankles my nerves when someone will say, "Oh, can't be too bad, after all, I'd like a weekly massage." They are probably thinking of a relaxing event, not a deep tissue torturous event. I hate to mention how painful it can be, one, because people don't believe me, and two, because people don't embrace painful events, even if they are therapeutic.

I think athletes led the way to making the general public understand the benefits of massage and ice baths. After all, their body is their office, their livelihood, it needs to be in top performance conditioning.

About 20 years ago, I was seeing a massage therapist who traveled with a well-known professional golfer. I lived in an area where there were big PGA tournaments. This massage therapist had a network of followers who would meet him at his hotel, and he would do body work. This network came from tennis players and professionals that I knew because I was playing competitive tennis in those days.

This gentleman changed my mind about massage. I was already a believer, but more for the comfort it gave me, not for the diagnosis it could provide. When I first met him, I was scheduled to have rotator cuff surgery.

I had attended a forum on shoulders, which is a very tricky body part because it is the nexus of the neck, arm, and back. At this forum there was a lady who kept coming back for years wanting shoulder surgery. The doctors kept telling her she had tendinitis or bursitis of the shoulder, not a tear which needed surgery.

With this story in the back of my head, I went to see this therapist named Jim. He worked on my shoulder and confirmed I needed surgery. He told me so many people get confused between lactic acid build up in a joint and real malfunctioning problems. I took his words to heart. To this day, I have kept up massage therapy once a week. A lady comes to my house. Expensive, but worth it for me.

MEDICATION

At first you start with over-the-counter medicines (OTC) like Tylenol, Advil, Aleve, Motrin, or Aspirin. They will help for a time, until they won't. Then the doctor will give you muscle relaxants. Those, too, will work a while and then they won't. Then you move to NSAIDs which are nonsteroidal anti-inflammatory drugs which are meant to address the inflammation and swelling which is compromising your body's ability to move. Think of swelling as a hot air balloon you'd like to deflate, settle you back to the ground instead of lifting you into the pain sectors.

For me, the real game changer was fifteen years ago when a woman I met came up to me at a party and said she could see I was in a lot of pain. Some people notice things like that. I explained I was but I distrusted the pharmaceutical industry because of the drug I had taken that messed up my eyes. She handed me a marijuana brownie and said, "Eat this tonight, and I believe you will get some relief." And I slept!!!

It was a godsend and to this day I think of her with great affection. The irony is, I used to be a counselor for teenagers getting out of drug rehab. I did not use marijuana in college or use it recreationally like many people did. I had a deceased husband who had drug addiction issues, and I was of the age when the War on Drugs was serious business. My children had gone through the Drug Abuse Resistance Education (DARE) programs in school. It was a leap of faith for me to embrace medicinal marijuana, but I am grateful I made the leap.

When I was a therapist, the teenagers I worked with came out of rehab with an addiction to nicotine, which was a transitional drug and one which calmed their nerves. I had no idea at the time that I would later find that illegal substance, marijuana, the most helpful pain fighting drug I ever used. I am so grateful to this day that I made this choice instead of narcotics.

As for nicotine, which is the most addictive drug there is, I never told my 12 charges out of drug rehab to stop smoking. However, at the end of a year working with them, I am pleased to report most of them had quit smoking.

The beauty of marijuana, unlike nicotine, is it reduces pain and won't cause any ill side-effects like cancer. You will not overdose, because if you take too much you will probably fall asleep and isn't that what we are hoping for? A little rest.

The trick is to learn how to use it. We are all individuals and it will impact us in a unique way. There isn't a "one pill" or "silver bullet" to this process. You must engage in your own healing.

In the early days, it wasn't legal. I am not a smoker, so I had to buy the product from nefarious sources or enterprising entrepreneurs, however, you choose to interpret it. I would make teas, cookies, and butters. I used a crockpot and if I lit a candle, the other residents in my apartment building couldn't smell it brewing.

Of course, nowadays, it is legal in many states. Fortunately, I live in such a place. So, if you are interested in exploring the pain-relieving qualities of marijuana, get thee to a dispensary.

You will be instructed there are two different strains of marijuana, Sativa and Indica. Sativa is fashioned for a psychotropic high which will affect mood and behavior – being BUZZED is often a description. Indica is for pain relief. I'll discuss Pain later, but I hope many of you can overcome your fear of marijuana and embrace its medicinal qualities. It is my go-to pain reliever.

MEDITATION AND MINDFULNESS

Meditation was something I think I came upon early in life although I didn't have a name for the process. I was the girl in the tree spending endless hours waiting for her father. While in that tree, I got into a transcendent place (I realize this looking back) where time, temperature, and traffic were irrelevant. I didn't even look at the cars going by on our seldom-traveled street. I was able to be at peace.

Later in my life, I watched the interviews between Bill Moyers and Joseph Campbell. Joseph Campbell was the author of "The Power of Myth" and was the man who coined the phrase, "follow your bliss". It was the New Age Wave that was forming in our country.

He addressed the issue of meditation explaining that it is a state of mind, not necessarily someone sitting in the lotus position going OOM, but gardening, swimming, walking in nature – all these activities are a form of meditation.

When I was able, I did those activities to calm my spirit. However, as my disease progressed and I needed surgery after surgery, I needed a different way to access that mind space.

I read a book by John Gray, the man who wrote "Men Are From Mars, Women Are From Venus." I don't remember which of his books I was reading, and when I looked at the volume of work he has done, I got flustered because I couldn't remember the title.

Essentially, he was suggesting you can meditate anywhere, any time. His mantra is, "Oh dear ___(insert whatever deity you worship) please come sit in my heart. I open my heart to you." I have used this while waiting for surgery, doctor's appointments, in airports. Any time I want to transport my mind and spirit away from the present situation.

I have since been instructed in Transcendental Meditation and practice that every morning. For years I didn't think I could fathom traditional meditation because I had gone to a class where everyone had to sit in the lotus position. This I could not do. I got frustrated with the instructor's insistence I really could do it if I wanted to, right? Mind over matter.

My back hadn't been fused by then, and it was agony for me to sit in that position. The instructor's intractable attitude turned me off. I knew him from Graduate School and he had an institute. Charged a lot. Was a guru. Never saw a guru again.

Nowadays, I lie in bed and meditate. I do some deep breathing, say my mantra, and voila! It is a smooth transition, no sitting in agonizing positions, just entering that magical space where you transcend the mind and body and enter the presence of the spirit, a very beautiful and pleasant universe.

This is sometimes hard to accomplish because pain can interfere with the transition of focus from the brain to the spirit. Your body is screaming, "FIRE IN THE HOLE!! What are you doing just lying there? Do something." Depending on your pain level, a topic discussed under P, you might be able to supersede the pain, or you might have to tough it out and meditate later. Maybe some stretching, soaking in a tub. My mantra with pain is, "I want to meditate, not agitate."

Mindfulness is a word often used, but I fear little understood. It is the consideration of how your words impact other people. Being aware of what comments or judgments are made can really soothe or exacerbate a situation. A kind comment can soothe, a cruel one can make people defensive and angry.

The four tenets of mindfulness are:

Non-judgment, Acceptance, Curiosity, and Compassion.

Perhaps this movement had more steam before Covid, because I don't often meet people in public who have embraced this way of being. It seems rude and bullish people are predominant these days. Nonetheless, I will soldier on and hope the trend becomes the norm.

For me, I have learned the following mind sets: Integrated, Logical, Emotional. When I am in pain, I am usually in an emotional brain. Too many surgeries make for too many painful memories, so I try to coax myself up the ladder – trying to access that logical brain station where I can make sense of everything. But my logical brain gets that none of this makes any sense, and then I pop up into integrated brain where I can accept the cold light of reality.

This is a rather loose and loopy description of a very important practice, but I know there are books written about this process, and this book is about Disability, so I hope you can investigate it. Mindfulness is incredibly liberating.

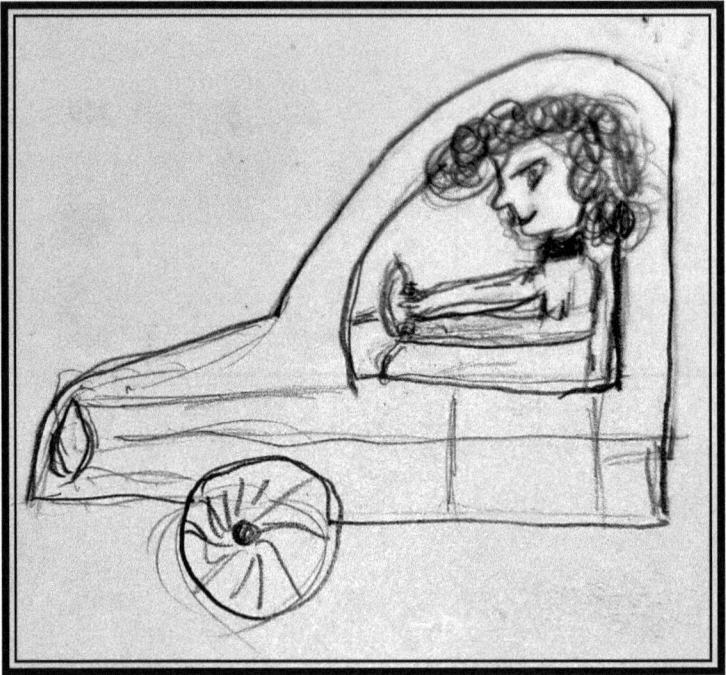

NERVES

Nerves and muscles work together. It's how we move around. It is called the neuromuscular system. Every move you make is because your muscles and nerves are working in concert.

So, when the muscles or nerves get strained or pinched, there is a painful reaction and a constriction of movement.

The interesting thing about nerves is we all think they are

emotional. "You are getting on my nerves". Or one has a nervous breakdown.

The problem with nerves is that they are players in both the physical and emotional worlds. Taking deep breaths and counting to ten can calm an angry person down. Taking deep breaths and focusing on the wounded body part can also bring relief.

When I was first hospitalized way back in 1978, the thought was that the nerve that connected to the digestive function of my body was being squished by a crumbled vertebrae in my neck.

The solution, in those days, was a neck brace and traction. So, I hung myself from a door jamb – one sits in a chair in the doorway with a strap or harness under the chin. It is a pulley system. Your neck on one side of the pulley, and a sandbag on the other. I am not even sure if they do that anymore because I can honestly say it wasn't that effective. I later segued into a unit where I could lay on the floor. Do that 30 minutes a day and the hope was it would relieve pain. All it did, after 10 years of faithful compliance, was to give me a Military Neck – over straightened.

The neck brace part was prescribed in the hospital with the caveat I must wear it whenever I was at risk. Riding horses, playing tennis, playing softball, and driving cars were all risky business, so I wore my cumbersome neck brace from 1978-2018 which was forty years of looking like a dork.

Sometimes, even when you do the right thing, it doesn't produce the expected result. Most doctors blame the patient. I just wish they'd admit the inefficiency and infancy of our medical system.

NURSING HOMES

This is a very personal category for me. The year was 1988 and I got a call from my stepmother. She was sending my 85-year-old father to me in an ambulance because he had been acting erratically for a few years, which we all knew, but now he had contracted pneumonia and she didn't want to deal with it. She had attached a note to him, "He's your father, you take care of him."

I loved my father, so I willingly embraced the task of his care. Nobody wanted to say he had Alzheimer's, so they insisted I call it senility. Whatever one wants to label it, it's a problem. The main problem is you are witness to the denigration of the human mind. His body, once we got over the pneumonia, was relatively strong.

I needed to find a nursing facility. My father was a wealthy man, so I decided to go for the best. In those years, it was $9,000 a month. In today's dollars with cost of living and inflation, it would be $24,000 a month.

I envisioned my father would get good care – like a 5-star hotel. Sad to say, not so much. I couldn't stay with him every day because I had two toddlers, a senior in high school, and a very troubled husband. So, I popped in when I could.

Early days were the worst, he wanted to go home. I wish I could have taken him home, but mine was not possible because of the chaos of toddlers, a teenager, and a crazy man.

My father was in a stylish, clean environment, and I knew he just needed to transition. I would go to meals with him in the evening when I could. At that time, he could feed himself and communicate with the other residents. He had been a Lieutenant Commander in the Navy during World War II, so he came up with the notion he was in the Officer's Club. Really helped him to calm down.

One time, I came not at mealtime and found him tied to a gurney with restraints. Trapped and frantic, my father fought because he was an officer and a gentleman, not someone who needed restraint. They tried to convince me it was for his own safety, and I get that part. However, it was not what I wanted for my father. I hired a companion, someone who sat with him from 9 in the morning until bedtime. It made a world of difference. I knew he had a protector.

It makes me so sad there aren't higher standards in nursing homes. A little-known fact is that 70% of nursing homes are run for profit, which is why they pay minimum wages to very underpaid, overworked employees. Got to get the profit to the investors. Anyone who has put a loved one in such a facility feels dreadful. The equivalent of leaving a dog at the pound. I believe taking care of people challenged with aging or illness or disability should be something to embrace, not something to shove out of sight lest we be reminded of their presence.

As I said, this is a very personal subject. When my brother was dying, I promised him he could die at home. He had seen the treatment my father had been given, and it frightened him.

The end of life can be so frightful for many people, I wish we could put more mercy into this world so upon leaving it, the inevitability of death could be seen as a transition, not a Grim Reaper event.

NUTRITION

You are probably thinking I covered this under diet, but it is a subject that needs to be hammered home because it is the foundation of wellness. You are what you eat is not a joke or a catchy diet phrase, it is literally the most important thing you can do for your body and wellbeing.

From an orthopedic point of view, excess weight and ill-conditioning put a tremendous stress on your body. I once heard every 5 pounds of extra weight on your frame carries a commensurate level of pressure not only to your joints, but also your heart. It has to work over time when you decide to lumber in an unfit body, rather than glide in a conditioned one. Your gait will be better, your heart will be lighter. It's a win-win.

Your heart and your stomach are the most dynamic organs in your body. ***Interestingly, heart disease is the leading cause of death in both men and women. It's really important to keep it as healthy as possible because it's keeping you alive.*** The heart is the big pumper of blood, but the stomach is more than a digestive cauldron, it is considered by some physicians to be the second brain.

My stomach is always the whistle blower of my bodily

functions. My original diagnosis back in 1978 was because of unremitting projectile vomiting. Listen to your stomach and feed it well. If you follow a good, healthy eating regimen, your heart and stomach will reward you with a longer, healthier life.

I started my nutritional quest in 1978, it is now 2025, and I am so grateful I chose the path I did. I do not have collateral damage from my disease – no diabetes, heart disease, obesity – I am fit in mind, if not body. You are your body's caretaker so try to embrace the power of your determination rather than a resignation that nothing can change. Nothing will change unless you take the reins of your health in your own hands and get to work.

O

OLD SCHOOL DOCTORS

My biggest problem with today's medical world is I remember the good old days when medicine was meant to be merciful, not mechanical. I loved the Dr. Welby days when your doctor was almost an extension of the family.

When my mother was so sick in the 1950s a doctor would often come to our house to visit her. Her doctor resembled Vincent Price, he was frightening to my child-like mind. I was told to stay out of the way. No problem. My brother and I would huddle under the piano and try to figure out what was happening. That was our go-to meet up place.

As I look back, I am so grateful she had that kind of attention. In today's medicine, many doctors, more often than not, are looking at their computer, not the patient. Surgeons have to look at you because they will touch you and ask where it hurts. The primary care doctors I've found are just looking at the numbers. Forget the person sitting in front of you – so, so sad. We've lost the human touch.

I count myself incredibly lucky that I now have a good team of doctors. My rheumatologist actually lives in another city. My daughter and I moved during Covid. Regardless, my rheumatologist has kept up with me, monthly visits for 4 years. My rheumatologist has been spot on in ordering ablations, trigger point injections, etc. I am so grateful for this doctor. In 2018 I had my first office visit. My hands and feet were in extreme pain. My hands were so swollen and inflamed I could not paint, which was the main enterprise I cared about. I was diagnosed with Psoriatic Arthritis. There is a monthly injection that can ameliorate the destruction of this disease. However, that injection was $1,500 back in 2018, probably more now. I couldn't afford it. My insurance wouldn't pay for it, probably because I had Medicare. If I'd had my daughter's insurance it would have been $50 a month. My very compassionate and competent physician gave me the shots for free, with the explanation the office got free samples once a month. This went on for almost a year. That beautiful doctor saved my hands allowing me to write this book today.

More currently, I have a pain doctor in the city where I presently live. It was just before Christmas, I had had to change practices from the former pain doctor because of extraordinarily uncomfortable chairs his patients were forced to endure. The reasoning given to me by the staff was that his wife was a decorator, and they wanted the right look. That did not fly with me. Appearance over health, really?

Luckily, I got in with a new group, but I was afraid I wouldn't be able to get the ablation in time to enjoy the Christmas holidays with my 29-year-old grandson. The new, compassionate doctor ordered an ablation, which is the burning of the nerves on the affected pain spot on your spine. Mine has always been my neck. I was so grateful. I had the best holiday.

Months later, I got a letter from an independent company saying the insurance would not pay for that ablation. My heart sank. The doctor had gone to bat for me, and now I probably need to pay up. I called his office, got the billing department, and I told the woman on the phone about the letter I had received. She said, "We will just have to eat it." I said, "What?" I couldn't believe it. I know there are so many rules and regulations about administering pain-saving procedures because, after all, aren't there just too many people with back problems or pain problems? At least that is the attitude I had often gotten in the past. I am so grateful to this pain doctor and my rheumatologists. It renews my faith in physicians.

I was listening to an interview with a brilliant man named Bessel van der Kolk, M.D., the author of "The Body Keeps the Score" the ground-breaking book on trauma and the effects on the body. This man lives in a large metropolitan area but chooses to go to a rural physician. He wanted a doctor who would take the time to talk to him and know him. For me, this is the essential missing part of modern medicine, the human touch.

Where I live now, there are concierge doctors. That is supposed to be a throw-back to a doctor who has time to attend to you, the doctor doesn't have an unbearable patient load. I wish I had had good success with this, unfortunately I did not. Again, the doctor was looking at the computer during most of our visits and did not take the time to get to know me. Now, I have found a new doctor, and I have high hopes. At least she looks at me.

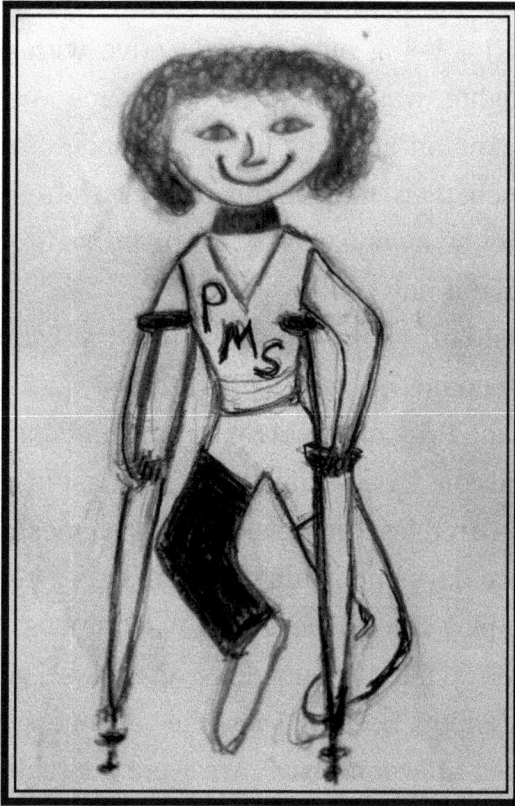

OPERATIONS

As I mentioned earlier, I have had 17 orthopedic and spinal surgeries. There is a list of them in the appendix. My first surgery was the only one caused by an accident resulting from injury rather than degeneration.

It was the first day of summer 1980. I had rallied my employees and friends to form a female softball team. For me, it was just what I wanted – being outside and active with people I care about. My daughter was our ball girl, our coach was a friend from high school, now an attorney married to one of our nurses. It was a fun bunch, there to have fun and be carefree. All of us had demanding jobs so no one was out for blood, so to speak, we saw that enough in our day jobs.

We had red ball caps with the letters PMS stamped across the top. My company was called Physicians Management Services and the Premenstrual Syndrome had not yet come into the popular jargon. Ever valiant were we. Last in the league but couldn't have cared less. We loved having picnics with our families on practice days and going to sports bars after game days.

I chose to play catcher because I was the boss and I knew I would get diverted if in the outfield or on a base. I get bored when there isn't any action. Besides, I was the only one who had an arm to throw an out at second base. We were adorable but not very competitive, we were just trying to have fun. Sadly, there are those who play sports to have fun, then there are those who must WIN.

Such was the case on the first day of summer in 1980. I was the ever-valiant catcher when there was a play at home plate. Our opponents had obviously chosen to play below their skill level. They came equipped with equipment bags, gloves, tattoos (not common in 1980), and a hard-core attitude.

So, in comes the ball from wherever, and I catch it. Simultaneously, one of the larger ladies (they were all larger than we were) plowed into me, clipped me at the knees and blew out my knee.

The injury wasn't as obviously alarming or attended to as it would be now with all our knowledge about ACL's, etc. It was the night of an important fight, Leon Spinks and someone else. My coach was a bit tipsy and didn't get in the face of the umpire like I wish he would have.

I went home, tried to soak it, then realized my knee was really messed up.

Sure enough, I needed surgery.

When I woke up in the hospital after anesthesia, I could not lift my head off the pillow because the discs in my neck were too weak to hold up my head. Eventually, I could lift my head, but anesthesia was to be my nemesis time after time post surgically.

Moreover, the surgeon who operated told me I had genetically weak knees and I would one day have serious problems if I didn't keep up my swimming – he knew I swam. We went to the same YMCA. His advice helped because it was almost 15 years before I needed any surgical intervention.

I think one of the hardest decisions is whether to operate now or later. Sometimes there isn't a choice. Now that I have artificial joints in all but one shoulder, I would like to sing from the rooftops, THEY ARE A MIRACLE! But if I had been afraid of having an operation, then I would definitely be wheelchair-bound today.

New Reno firm helps doctors run their offices

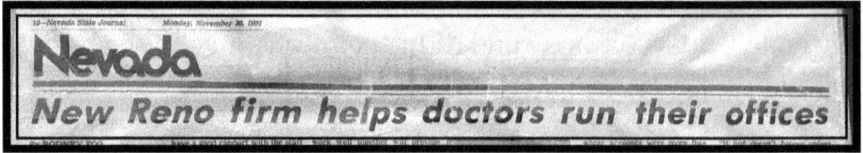

OPPORTUNITY COSTS

It is difficult to tally what disability costs. Is the bottom line impact on the GNP? Is it the missed work, all those missed appointments?

For me, it was the opportunity cost of continuing in a profession I was well-suited and well-trained for.

I don't need to bang on about how I was 29 when this hit me, so trust me when I tell you, there have been intrinsic costs plus the very real loss of a livelihood. For me, I was fortunate that I was able to sell my business, and that coupled with an inheritance from my parents, allowed me to sustain a very comfortable lifestyle. Having an MBA helped to manage money and investments. I am so overwhelmingly grateful.

Such is not the case for many disabled souls. You see them on the streets and in homeless camps. Non-functioning body parts are rarely a source of enterprise, unless you're Franklin Delano Roosevelt or Stephen Hawking or a king, like Richard III.

Actually, quite a few celebrities have been unashamed of their disabilities and have become public role models.

Here's a list of 10 celebrities who have been open about their disabilities.

1. **Stephen Hawking** – Physicist, had ALS, which caused progressive paralysis.
2. **Helen Keller** – Author and activist, was both deaf and blind.
3. **Michael J. Fox** – Actor, has Parkinson's disease.
4. **Selma Blair** – Actress, diagnosed with multiple sclerosis.
5. **Franklin D. Roosevelt** – Former U.S. President, had polio and used a wheelchair.
6. **Stevie Wonder** – Musician, blind since birth.
7. **Christy Brown** – Writer and painter, had cerebral palsy, wrote "My Left Foot."
8. **Halle Berry** – Actress, has type 1 diabetes.
9. **Daniel Radcliffe** – Actor, has dyspraxia, a developmental coordination disorder.
10. **Marlee Matlin** – Actress, deaf since childhood

This is probably not an exhaustive sample of celebrities who have had challenges. It happens no matter how rich and famous you are.

PAIN

This is the granddaddy of all topics for me. The defining force that has shaped my life. The tricky problem with disabilities is that not all of them are painful. Mine happens to be, so I consider myself an expert of pain.

I have been hospitalized twice with pain so intense, I could scarcely stand or walk.

Being admitted for pain, I got a lot of attitude from the staff with comments like if you'd just think happy thoughts, or it's really not that bad, or some foolishness like that. Let me tell you when you can't walk, it really is that bad.

Those admittances to the hospital were over twenty years ago. Not only have I had corrective surgeries, but there is a more enlightened attitude about pain.

In the early days of my disease, there were no doctors practicing pain management. In hospitals, there were physiatrists (PM&R doctors). PM&R (Physical Medicine and Rehabilitation) was established in 1933. They were mainly hospital-based because the physical effects of pain were just starting to be understood.

What helped punctuate the need for these physiatrists were the war wounded returning home after World War II. The marvel of military wounds stills my heart because the soldier's level of suffering has to be off the charts. I think of the battle amputations during the wars where no ambulances were around to carry the war-wounded to safety. How did they manage the pain?

When my first child was born, my husband was serving in the military during the Vietnam War. My daughter was born in a military hospital. After 15 hours of a rough labor, there was concern that my baby was stuck. I was taken to x-ray in the middle of the night.

The middle of the night was when the war wounded were treated because any sight of their injuries would be extremely upsetting to other dependents coming into the hospital during the day. I find it sad that they could not be seen in the light of day. Too scary.

When I was rolled into x-ray, I saw young men with gaping, horrific wounds. It was heart wrenching. There I was having a baby, looking at 18-year-old boys serving their country who had holes in their stomachs, missing jaws, and missing limbs. It was so harrowing. I have never forgotten their faces. When there is talk of wounded warriors, we must remember how they sacrificed their well-being for our safety. It troubles me deeply that we treat them so shabbily and question their valor.

For many years, I dealt with the pain of my disease, but finally it got too much. I first met a physiatrist in 2005 when my back was causing me all kinds of trouble. I was given trigger point injections. Any relief is welcome relief, even if it doesn't erase the pain. I was so gratified someone helped me with my pain instead of shaming me for my pain.

In 2006, I met my first real pain doctor. He was one of the most compassionate and competent doctors I have ever met. It was then I discovered the miracle of the ablation, a procedure where the nerves are burned – in this case in my neck. They would provide almost immediate relief, often resulting in swelling along the neck and spinal cord creating more pain for a week or so. Knowing pain will go away someday is music to the ears of a chronic pain sufferer. A week of discomfort knowing I will be pain-free for a few months was a price I was willing to pay.

This is when I was introduced to the Pain Scale. Developed in 1975 by Dr. Ronald Melzack and Dr. Warren Torgerson at McGill University, it is now considered a vital sign.

The way I interpret the pain scale on a 1-10 is I make it about percentages. If you're in level 1, then ten percent of your body is diverted, reacting to the pain. If you're in level 2, 20 percent, – so on and so forth. I like to describe it this way because a person at level 6 has 60% of their body, mind, and spirit fighting to stay calm and carry on.

Chronic pain is that enduring pain that just doesn't go away with seemingly routine injuries. Let's say you stubbed your toe. Tricky to walk, but you know if you're careful it will subside and you can walk normally.

Chronic pain is the condition where the pain never subsides, or so intermittently or unpredictably that the sufferer never feels safe. Will I be able to go out and be with friends without being a big, old bucket of pain?

For many years, my running level of pain was about 5, and that was a good day.

Let me explain – the pain scale is from 1-10:

1 – almost no sensation of pain or so minor it doesn't disturb you - perhaps a minor bruise.

2 – a little more pain, but nothing to divert your attention and take your day away, like a paper cut.

3 – this is when you start to notice something. Perhaps a mild headache or tightness in a muscle.

4 – it is at this level where you might seek medical intervention or take medication because it is annoying enough to seek help.

5 – This is going to throw a wicket in your day. It will be hard to get out of bed, move around. Muscle relaxants and NSAIDs will probably be recommended but they come with their own bag of side effect tricks.

6 – is when they bring in the pain fighting department – opioids or narcotics. This is the level where people can get truly messed up if they do the wrong thing or the doctor prescribes some medication that is, trust me, going to play havoc on your stomach. It is the level that takes you out of the game.

7 – is the level that takes you off the playing field completely. For me, level 7 means hospitalization, usually. I need intervention because it is very difficult to walk and my stomach is roiling so I have dry heaves with every step I take. I have been in the ER twice at a level 7 and have gotten pain relieving injections that went directly into my skull right to the brain. What a relief! Life becomes bearable. Since I have had my 17 surgeries, I have not experienced level 7, and for this, the surgeries have been a blessing.

8 – another rung on the pain ladder but has only come to me post-operatively while I am still in the hospital. It is the level where you can still talk, and you can breathe on your own, but the misery is crushing.

9 – is where I can no longer communicate. I call it my Blink and Breathe level because that is all you can do. In fact, one is often put on oxygen at this

level because your body has all systems on deck for the pain, not the other daily functions it performs, like breathing.

Level 10 – I am truly not sure I've gone to the top of the scale, but 9 was relatively close.

I have read so many pithy articles, like "Let Pain be Your Teacher" which annoyed me. Okay, if you want a miserable and abusive teacher. I have overcome my pain issues, but am very aware, they can resurface any day of the week and they sometimes do. Chronic pain people are known for good days and bad days, trust me, they are real.

When I go to the doctor and they ask for my pain level, I get confused sometimes. I might have a level 4 pain in my ankle, a level 6 pain in my neck, and a level 3 in my back. Of course, it depends on what doctor I am seeing, but if I explain all those different body parts that are in pain, sometimes I get the eye roll of intolerance, like just keep it simple, please. But pain isn't simple, it's insidious.

However, I have new hope. Recently, I saw a *TED Talk* with Kim Baxter, who is a physician, and her talk title was "How to Hack Your Brain When You're in Pain." She uses ice and vibration to disrupt the running of the pain zooming 200 MPH around your body. It is brilliant, and I recommend it to you all.

Please acknowledge, people without pain problems, that pain is real and can often manifest in pain brain. I mentioned casually that pain travels at 200 MPH around your body. The genesis of the pain is your brain. That is where the term "pain brain" applies. Your mind cannot grasp details because it is fighting a battle in your body. I have had a lot of years with foggy thinking and multiple failures of judgment, but now, gratefully, my brain is back in focus. It is a precious thing to feel able to think after so many pain-ridden years, but it isn't smooth sailing.

For most of this book, I have written when I was not above a level 4 in pain, but lately, I have been battling a persistent level 6 in my neck. In the last 10 days, I have spent 3 of them in bed, unable to do my regular routine. Mostly, it throws me back when I have to go to bed and stay there – back to the long years of surgery and convalescence.

However, I have figured out the trigger. I was trying to interact and be social. I tried to play Bridge with a group on Saturday mornings. No problem, right? Well, the first problem was my eyes which couldn't handle the fluorescent lights and the fans, which the organizers fixed by putting my table in a very shady area. So I went back full of bravado, I can go out, I can be social. Sadly, I realize it wasn't just my eyes protesting, but now my back wasn't happy with my sitting. Sitting to type a book and sitting to play Bridge are not compatible. I have had to suspend Bridge until I am recovered and no longer need to sit to write. In other words, I need to isolate myself.

I bring this tale of woe to you because I want you to understand that having chronic pain means it NEVER goes away. I can mitigate it with shots, ablations, marijuana, massages, stretching, and heat therapy, but I cannot conquer it. I have learned to co-exist with my pain days and have very limited and controlled social interactions. Pain is truly a four-letter word.

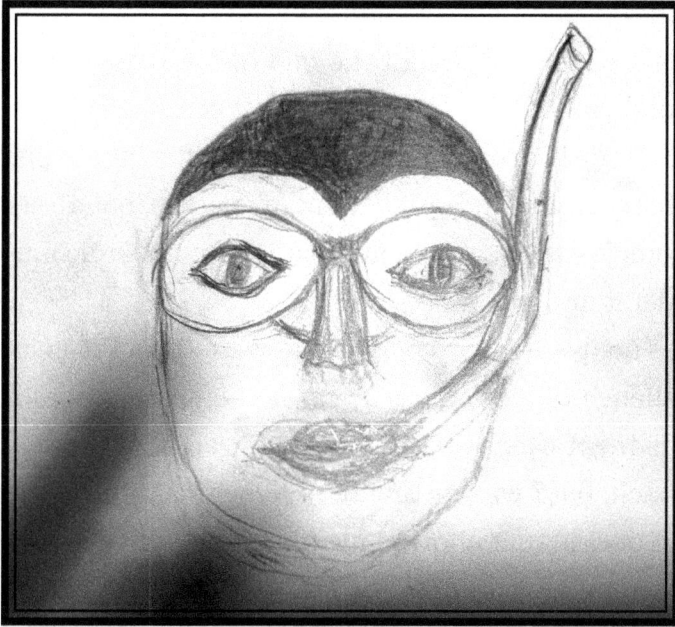

PERSISTANCE

I originally titled this category as PARALYMPICS because to me, they are the epitome of people who have persisted through pain and injury. However, I never watch the Paralympics, so it felt a bit disingenuous. I have enormous respect for these athletes because their work ethic and fortitude to overcome whatever obstacle kept them out of the game are admirable beyond measure.

This is where my angst surfaces, because I have the discipline and dedication of an athlete, but my body will prevent me from playing the game. The lady in the sauna comes to mind. Someone who could swim, and I couldn't. Outside looking in has never been comfortable for me. At the end of the day, I am armchair bound and can only watch them play, it is a space denied to me and I find it disheartening to face my own inability to perform.

Perhaps that sounds petty to many people, but after reading my chronicles with surgery and pain, I am hopeful some of you can understand.

I was so desperate to play in the water that I once accepted the challenge of a very stern and non-empathic person to try scuba diving. I was worried about the weight of the scuba tank on my back, but I was fortunate to be with a forgiving and kind group of people that allowed me to suit up with the tank once I had gotten in the water.

It was a marvelous sense of freedom. I had been an ocean swimmer before, and it was like coming home. Like all homes, there are mixed messages – because there are inherent dangers – sharks, sting rays, eels, that sort of thing.

Apprehension and excitement co-exist in so many athletic disciplines which is what makes them so rewarding and exciting. To conquer the unknown, the thrill of accomplishment, these are heady rewards for risk.

Ocean swimming is an unpredictable place which is half the challenge. Otherwise, swim in a pool if you want to be on the safe side. I was an ocean swimmer who used to be more full of adventure.

The ocean water I had swam in for many years was crystal clear and I loved it! Besides swimming in the ocean, I loved snorkeling and about 12 years ago tried scuba diving. I was slightly disoriented after my ocean swimming days, I was in a different ocean environment. I didn't see as many colorful fishes but I saw octopus and turtles and tuna. Sadly, my scuba life was a short-lived freedom.

On my last trip, I got back to the boat where I had to hoist myself up the ladder to get inside. For 3 outings, my shoulder had no complaint. On the 4th outing, my already-operated-on shoulder glitched and I knew I would need a rotator cuff repair.

I didn't see this complication coming when I tried that sport, but perhaps I should have. It's hard to know what tolerance your body parts want when you have a heart for adventure, but I had a very fragile body held together by bailing wire and metal joints. I am wiser these days, I know, but then I still hoped and hope can be so dangerously dashed.

I mention the Paralympics because as much as I admire their courage and competitive nature, I knew my courage and competitive nature had to be homebound. No work outs, games, or travel allowed. No more going off book.

A few years ago, I became aware of Suleika Jaouad, a beautiful young woman who contracted Leukemia when she was in her early 20s, which would require years of hospitalization. She turned her pain and distress into action, and wrote a column for the New York Times called "A Life Interrupted" about her struggle with chemotherapy and bone marrow transplants. She wrote a book called *Between Two Kingdoms* – a personal description of the divergent worlds of the vigorous and healthy versus the struggling chaos of disease and disability. When I read her book, it jumped into my psyche. Her bravery and perseverance are incredibly inspiring. I recommend it to anyone who is feeling sorry for themselves in the chaos of disease and disability.

—————

PHYSICAL THERAPY

The most impressive gain, to me, in the management of orthopedic injuries is physical therapy.

Back in the 70s when I was first diagnosed with DDD (Degenerative Disc Disease), physical therapy was never mentioned. I was athletic and swam through most of my recoveries, until I couldn't swim because of shoulder and spinal surgeries. I still tried water exercise, but it wasn't enough.

Physical therapy came to my attention as a viable healing modality in the 1990s when physical therapists were now a part of my treatment team, providing healing spaces to focus on my hip, and later my knees, then my shoulders, then my neck, then my back, then my hands. Prior to 1990, I don't remember physical therapists being so important, but as I am a multi-faceted patient, I have come to appreciate them and rely on their knowledge and wisdom.

I think the old-time major misconception was that if you had an injury, don't move it. Isolate it. Remember all those casts you used to see? Encase the injury and give it time to heal. The time to heal part was important, but the isolation was misguided and created other unforeseen problems, like bone loss.

Physical therapy today has four modalities: stretching the body, strengthening the body, massage, and heat or ice therapy.

It is hard to do any of those treatments with a body part encased in a cast.

Stretching is self-explanatory – we all need to stretch, especially seniors. By doing so, we open our bodies to the proper blood flow by un-bunching aging muscles. For many years, stretching was the most underrated and ignored aspect of maintaining structural health. The popularity of yoga and Pilates has certainly addressed this issue and has provided benefits to both physical health and mental health. Love your body, nurture your spirit.

Strengthening is a bit trickier. When recovering from an injury, we often don't know when to challenge our body and when to protect it. Thankfully, the physical therapist can be your coach to put you back in the game, hopefully, with no recurrence of injury. Professional sports have led the way, from my point of view, because time is money and if a player can't suit up, that means money is lost, and the game will be lost, and the fans will be pissed off. Fitness has become the hallmark of champions – no more Babe Ruth's with explosive talent but a neglected body.

Massage became more acceptable and understandable thanks to physical therapy. I grew up in a generation where touching your own body was discouraged because of some sexual taboos, and I believe, for me, that extended to rubbing your own injured body part. Am I doing something harmful? Will it make it worse?

The maxim for heat or ice is, if it is a new injury, ice is where it's at. I developed a mantra, "Ice is Nice," because it truly is a miraculous relief. Freezing the area makes the pain slow down. Perhaps a more scientific explanation can be found, but for me, I craved ice treatments. A bit messy if you are bed-ridden, but completely worth the inconvenience.

Heat comes later. After the stitches have been removed, stiffness sets in. I favor infrared heat. I discovered this about four years ago and do an infrared treatment approximately 5 times a week. Because I am still trying to be active with water exercise and swimming, my body will get stiff and cranky. The infrared is a godsend. I recommend it to everyone.

I live in a desert so the temperatures are extreme. It is difficult to use the heat treatments in the summer when the temperatures are in triple digits and heat stress is a real concern. But in the winter, it is my cozy recovery place. It erases the aches and pains.

I think one of the impediments for people embracing physical therapy is that it causes pain, which is temporary and necessary, but when you have been through the surgical ringer or been compromised by an injury, the last thing you want is more pain. This is a difficult hurdle for some people. Again, athletes and military types get the necessity to endure temporary discomfort to get back on the road again, or as I refer to it, "back in the saddle again."

Puzzling, some people would prefer to be permanently on the DL (disabled list) because they don't see a way out. To me, this is the saddest thing of all. There is almost always a way out, if you know how to look for it and if you will seize the day and work on your body, mind, and spirit. It is a three-pronged effort, after all.

I had remarked earlier that I have recently gone through some physical therapy to regain the ability to climb stairs and to walk with a smoother gait. The process took about 6 months.

In this world of impatience, very few people will take the time to really rewire their bodies. I am old so I have plenty of time on my hands and prefer to use that time to get better, not sit around and complain.

Sometimes when I start the remodeling of my body, I get unexpected consequences. For example, I watched a YouTube channel on how to smooth your walking gait. YouTube has some wonderful resources to help rehabilitate injuries, and I have used it many times to treat different challenges.

This specific exercise had the patient standing on a step (like one used in aerobic classes) and stepping off with a weight in the hand of the side to which you are stepping. This works marvelously, by the way, but the unintended consequence was it challenged my right-arm bicep tendon and it was NOT happy. I have had four shoulder surgeries on my right arm, so I got the message and stopped that exercise. Gratefully, I think the exercise worked even after a brief time. No longer do people stop me on the street and ask if I need help, which is kind of them, but also points out my unsteady walking gait. For about 2 months now, I have had the ability to walk with less limping. I am no faster in my gait, but at least I am not so noticeably lame.

Physical therapy is an essential tool in your recovery plan. It will pay off in ways you cannot contemplate. Also, Medicare and most insurance plans pay well. My understanding is physical therapists are well-paid these days and worthy assets to your medical world.

Q

QUARRELSOME PEOPLE

Another phrase one might know is toxic people. These are the ones who come at you with their own agenda. My personal definition is they are the ones who make simple things complicated. If they are a caretaker, they may feel the need to restructure your day to try to motivate you with put-downs about being lazy or cheating or not trying hard enough. If not that direct, they might quarrel with you over the simple things – like what's for dinner or what tasks need to be accomplished. They want control of you, although they have no clue what is going on inside of you, they want to conduct your physical life, which is necessary, but can be done without much contentious banter.

You might have been raised with difficult people and take it for granted there will be complaints and criticisms constantly coming your way. Perhaps it is a pattern of communication you are comfortable with, but for me, the incessant bickering and debate are exhausting.

Different families communicate differently and we pick up those patterns in early childhood. I was raised in a Quaker-like house – no official church attendance, but a definite identification with their philosophies of austerity, pacifism, non-materialism, and non-commercialism. Our house was quiet, but not peaceful; organized, but not humanized; and it was never run for the benefit of the children, as so many homes are these days. So, quarrelsome people grate on my nerves – anywhere I encounter them.

About 20 years ago, I had a very difficult knee replacement. My daughters were away at university, so I needed to hire a caretaker. This woman whose name I cannot remember, which says a lot right there, came from an agency to help me. Anyway, this nameless caretaker took it upon herself to re-order my room. I didn't ask her to, I didn't want her to, and I kept asking her to leave things alone, which she did not. She kept bringing me orchids to "pretty up" my room. Orchids are gorgeous, so I knew what she was aiming for, but I didn't want them in my house, I had enough house plants, I didn't need more flora or fauna.

For her it was a decorative ornament, for me it was one more thing to take care of when I could barely walk. She couldn't clock my reasoning and persisted in this endeavor.

As hard as I would try to communicate with her, she would insist she was correct and I would feel "right as rain" if I just relaxed and soaked in the orchid's beauty.

To this day, I admire orchids, but I NEVER want to own one. It reminds me of how I had to quarrel with her about something she couldn't understand. She wanted control of my person and my environment.

I filter quarrelsome people out of my life whenever possible, and I am grateful my current family members are calm and caring.

Dealing with the disruption of other people's dysregulated personalities is taxing when you are focused on healing.

There are so many times we do not have a choice. In a

hospital, you really are flat on your back and have to take what you can get. But at home, you are vulnerable to the anxieties and overwhelm many caretakers and patients can experience together, rather like bringing a new baby home for the first time. It takes time to figure out what will work. If the bed is the right height, if trip hazards, like throw rugs, are out of the way. Lots of adjustments need to be considered.

If you come from a quiet household like I did, noise feels so invasive, and the noise of people arguing drives me to a level of agitation that isn't healthy for me.

For some people, bickering is their "love language". It is the only way they feel comfortable, like an amazing tennis match throwing barbs back and forth. But for the spectators (me) on the sidelines, it can be extremely agonizing.

I have stopped watching modern sitcoms and movies because I find the way people communicate in those settings is combative and aggressive.

Combative and aggressive is not a good healing space – peace and calm are much more helpful, at least for me. But I was born in the 1940s and the world was quieter then. Machines hadn't come to help us forget to be civil with each other.

There was a time when people gathered together and turned off their TVs or computers – nowadays, it seems like most people prefer looking at their phones instead of making eye contact. Even doctors will often stare at their computer and scarcely make eye contact, making me wonder why I even need to be there, we could have connected via computer or an audio visit.

Because we don't gather in social settings, except at church or the synagogue or the temple, I think we have forgotten how to care about other peoples' needs. The need to be listened to and understood, and hopefully not yelled at and lectured. That is my prayer, we learn to listen to each other with kindness instead of criticism.

QUESTIONS

Inevitably, when you are first diagnosed or fresh out of an accident or traumatic event, you have so many questions. Why me? What happened? When will I get better? Where will I be able to live?

The "Why Me?" part can be a complete stumbling block for some people. I know I was asking that when I was 29 years old and had my life in front of me. In the early days, I had no idea of the lengths arthritis would go to to disrupt my life, and I am grateful for that. If I had told my younger self I would have an excruciatingly painful disease that would require 17 surgeries, 10 years of being bedridden, and the loss of most of my pleasurable activities like walking, reading, swimming, driving a car, playing tennis, riding a horse, or just the simple act of sitting in a chair without discomfort, I probably wouldn't have believed it.

I am strong willed, and I want to overcome. There are just some battles you cannot win, and the sooner I accepted that, the easier my struggle became. I knew I couldn't overcome

Arthur, my arthritis nemesis, so I tried to find a way to coexist. But Arthur is an aggressive tyrant that wants to dominate and subjugate, not live in peaceful coexistence.

I am 76 now and looking back at the struggle of the last 47 years, I realize I did overcome. Not the physical aspects so much, but definitely the mental ones. I am not defined by my disease, but I cannot say I feel empowered by it. My limitations and pain keep me in the loop of never really feeling confident or comfortable in situations I cannot control, like chairs or lighting or bathroom accommodations. My degenerated eyesight keeps me out of places with fluorescent lights which prohibits me from playing bridge with a group of people I like very much.

Not sure Arthur was the culprit this time, but my genetics definitely are. My father had Macular Degeneration, therefore so do I. So, the "Why Me?" The answer is I had two parents, my mother's sister had a degenerative disease that landed her in a wheelchair by the time she was 40, and my father had Macular Degeneration which meant his golden years were spent sitting alone playing solitaire and watching sports on TV, no more reading his favorite books.

Nothing to be done but accept reality, but some people don't want to face the obvious and drone on and on about how unfair life is. Grow up. Nobody has it easy in this life, so why should you be any different?

The "What Happened?" question for me wasn't obvious when I was younger and hadn't had to face so many surgeries, but now, looking back, I realize it was a train wreck. What happened to me has been a torturous trial of surgery after surgery after surgery. I am so grateful I had competent surgeons because it could have turned out to be more of a disaster, and for this I am grateful.

What happened to you may not be your fault, as it was for me. Or maybe you were the cause of a car accident, or you were wounded in battle. What happened may be more obvious, but nonetheless, just as painful and debilitating. And then there are all those annoying questions, "What happened to you?" And people want to know, sometimes. I find with some people that if I try to explain what happened, their eyes glass over and they wait impatiently for me to finish. I think it would be more fun if I say I got hit by a truck on a snowy, snowy night. Something more dramatic, you know?

About ten years ago, I was in a major airport hanging out, like you do in airports. A beautiful woman walked by, and her companion who I assumed was her husband came behind her. He had lost both of his legs, he was skillfully rolling through the airport in one of those big wheeled contraptions like the Paralympians use, and he had a "get out of my way" attitude about him. It was an obvious battle wound because he had ARMY blazoned on his tee shirt. I am thinking that guy had to be an officer. He had an air of pride and command about him. The loss of his legs didn't seem to have diminished his will and spirit to strive. He had a beautiful wife, and I often look back and hope they are still together.

"When will I get better?" This is a toughie question to answer because there are so many variables. For my first knee replacement, I was completely naïve. In fact, my tennis partner had organized this sailing trip, and I was only a few weeks post-op. My doctor told me there was no way I should go on such an excursion, but again, I had knee surgeries in the past and thought I knew better, but a knee replacement is a whole sight different than a meniscus repair.

I showed up for the excursion, there were probably 15 people on the boat, and I was with my walker. I was in pain, no comfortable place to sit, and I was seething inside. Why didn't I listen to my doctor? Why does it take so long to heal?

My first knee replacement was in 2003. I think they have improved considerably in the last 21 years, but please be kind to yourself. It's going to take a minute for you to be back on your feet. I attribute some of my impatience to my youth. I was only 54 years old and I still had a lot of living to do, but it wasn't going to be the able-bodied life I had so enjoyed.

"Where will I be able to live?" This is a question on many an elderly person's mind, even if they are able-bodied. For the disabled, I pray they have resources, because besides the emotional costs to disability, it is expensive. If you can afford therapists, remodeling your home with ramps, guardrails, or showers for accessibility, then you are the lucky ones. I count myself in this category. I have had years of therapy, own my home, and I live alone.

If I did not own my own home or couldn't afford to live alone, then I would have very limited options, indeed. Sadly, some disabled people find themselves on the streets. I hate that we have homeless, but so very often, they are the disabled who cannot meet the demands of a work force life and don't have a financial base like I do.

I, myself, never wanted to go to a rehabilitation facility after my surgeries. I chose to go home, and perhaps my children would have preferred I had gone to rehab. I rarely do well in institutionalized settings, so I knew I wouldn't heal well with fluorescent lights and regimented meals and noise and human activity. When I am rehabbing, I never want a television blaring or people around me. I want to suffer in silence when it comes to my physicality.

We are all different, and I suggest that being challenged as I have been, will help you figure out who you are, what you can do, when you can take action, and where you can settle. I hope you have some choices, so few of us do.

QUIET

As I mentioned, I find peace and quiet essential to my own healing. Other people are different. I understand the roar of the crowd at a sporting event might divert you from the roaring going on in your painful body.

I do like diversion, but I want to control the parameters. I do not like violent or scary things. My disease has been violent and scary enough, thank you very much.

As I reflect on humanity's journey with understanding disease and disability, I realized there have been different concepts for how to help people.

In the early 1900s the scourge of tuberculosis was almost pandemic. The thought in those days was to remove patients from the chaos of the cities and move them to the comfort of the country. Fresh air and open spaces would provide an ease to living and breathing. The real antidote was antibiotics, but they were not discovered until 1928 so no help was on the horizon before then. Compassionately, sanitoriums were constructed to soothe the spirits of the suffering.

Eventually, tuberculosis became less of a scourge, then polio entered the scene, and it was highly contagious and wasn't under control until the poliovirus was discovered in 1949 and subsided in about 1979. When you think about it, it wasn't very long ago.

The mission for sanitoriums would segue into sanitariums – same concept, different reason. Peace and quiet for the returning war wounded would put them to rights and back to being productive. Or, people suffering nervous afflictions could find comfort in quietude. These were places like resort spas for the suffering. Lots of good food, exercise, consistent care, and quiet. The expense of running such places became astronomical, and the advent of modern hospitals reduced the need to travel. We had so much to learn back then, and we still do today.

A modern-day hospital is a beehive buzzing with the business of patient care, controlling infections, and so many more considerations than back in the 1900s. I often try to understand the despair they must have felt, but then I realized they were doing the best they could with the information they had. They didn't have televisions detailing every aspect of human existence, and not always in pleasant ways.

Knowledge is power, and we have so much more knowledge about disease and its causes, but I wonder if we are any better at understanding the healing process of human beings. This will be discussed under Trauma, but it is worthy of note here, because with the advent of the internet, we are perpetually bombarded with ad after ad, email after email, portal after portal, and apps popping up everyday.

It is a bit of mayhem, and it doesn't account for people who want peace and quiet. Oh, you can hire an assistant to run interference, but at the end of the day, it is you who will have to take care of so much of the business of living and healing.

Quiet is something I crave in those non-functional conditions. However, the world has just gotten noisier and noisier, and people shut themselves into their own worlds with headphones to escape the chaos. I have done this time after time in hospitals, dental offices, and waiting rooms. Loud TV's seem to be the norm in doctors' waiting rooms these days. What happened to reading a book? Being able to calmly wait your turn without the thump, thump, thump of loud music or ads.

I think this is why people are so wont to shut out the voices of strangers. They don't want to hear your problems, they just want the solace of whatever is blaring in their ears.

I wear ear plugs at the dentist because when my teeth are being cleaned or I have a procedure, the noise is agitating. Other people seem inured to it because I'll search whatever noisy space I'm in and wonder if they can't hear it, too? My phone even alerts me when I am in a loud environment. I suspect I have spent too much time in my own solitary world and find the outside world extremely noisy and chaotic.

I like the idea of sanitariums (sanitoriums is where TB patients went) because I find the best healing can happen in the calm and stillness of the eye of the storm, not battling all the challenges and congestions of city life. I prefer the country life, but I know many of my family would be bored out of their gourd with the bucolic quietude. Perhaps rehab would be the best option for them.

But for many who have been "shell-shocked," quiet is seductive to calm the nerves and get back in the game when we are healed and strong enough to take on modern life.

RECOVERY

Recovery is a tricky word. In health it isn't exactly like recovering a lost phone or lost personal item, it is more like trying to patch up Humpty Dumpty all the time. All the King's horses and all the King's men couldn't put him back together again, either.

Some surgeries and recoveries are less severe than others. With some surgeries, one can recover their former movement and activities. I imagine youth is more likely to find this than the elderly ones struggling to find balance because their life has been unbalanced.

The key to recovery is you. I know there are medical people who can help, even mental trainers can help your mind adjust to your new reality, but none of those people are going to help if you don't have the right mindset.

If you are stuck in the questions part and want answers NOW, the answer often is time will tell. Healing takes time, and in our fast-paced world of zoom, zoom professionals dominating the landscape, time to heal becomes a rare and precious commodity.

This was a lesson that came to me the hard way. If I tried to rush things, wham, I was slapped back down by shaky legs and wobbly arms. I was in the soup of sorrow trying to recover for about ten years.

I once clocked that in five years, I only woke up one time out of pain. I am not talking level three or four of annoying pain, I am talking massive, paralytic pain. I couldn't move until I had coaxed my body to rise up and get me to the bathroom, please.

Warm baths helped, but I had to give those up 10 years ago because I couldn't get myself out of a bathtub, something I tried to ameliorate by buying a walk-in tub. This is one of my more disappointing purchases on the road to recovery because it takes a long time to fill, and you'll need to get a new hot water tank because they are so large, the hot water runs out.

I paid for a new water heater system, I got myself bath salts and bubbles to enjoy the bliss of a good soak. It became a nightmare. I'd try to relax, but there is not a capability to recline, one must sit up. For a person with a fused spine, sitting up is a painful proposition. Fortunately, I sold the house where I had it installed, and the new owners were happy for it. If one doesn't have trouble sitting, I could see where it could be soothing, just not for me.

Recovery is a very long process after some especially complicated surgeries, like my cervical spine fusion. I mentioned earlier that I needed constant attention in the first two weeks of the acute recovery phase.

However, once my neck and throat started to heal, I found I could not eat certain things, like lettuce or apples. I love salads and I love apples, but I was basically on the boiled potatoes, apple sauce, and soft foods for almost a year.

Even now, some eight years later, I have trouble chewing

lettuce, so nowadays, I go for the chopped salads where the lettuce is pre-cut and more digestible.

I understand if a person doesn't have resources or referrals, their recovery may not be the outcome expected. They may not be "on the road again," they might be permanently stuck in their physical limitations. When I get stuck in this mindset when I am trying to get my leg to work, I am reminded of the lady in the sauna and have a clear realization that I do have a leg, and if I want it to work, what do I need to do?

We cannot rely on others to do the work for us. We must stretch, strengthen, massage, and ice ourselves to get better. Some of these efforts need other people to help, like the massage, but the stretching and strengthening part is following the game plan set by your physical therapist. Please follow their play book.

RESILIENCE

Of course, that is what it takes to fully recover, to have the resilience to jump through hurdles, and if you fall down, to get up and get back in the game of life.

For me, it wasn't the same game I had played in the past. No tennis, no long walks, no horseback riding, no driving a car, no ocean swimming, no reading my favorite books or poems – all testaments to the losses my disease had created. But there is a way to find joy after you are over the shock of the losses. I have learned how to manage debilitating pain, even though I suffer extreme pain more than I like. About 5 or 6 days a month, I will have to go down with a level 5 or 6 of pain. Nausea is the usual culprit, and it is nausea reminiscent of 47 years ago when I was hospitalized. I no longer vomit uncontrollably because I can lie down at home, I can find a way to control the pain. But if I am in public, it is extremely embarrassing to be retching at the early warning signs. Usually, it starts out as a level 6, and if I can keep it from climbing the pain charts, I can set myself to rights with quiet, soothing balms I put on my neck. Mostly, I need to completely withdraw from the world.

It is because of this propensity for the pain to strike when I least expect it that I don't get involved in many social obligations. People get their feelings hurt if I don't show up or decline invitations to parties or get-togethers.

This is an awkward space – after all, it's just a party, get out, you'll enjoy yourself talking to people and getting out of your own head. All these sentiments are meant kindly, but once they clock the limitations of my physicality, they back off. Trust me, I don't like being this no-show or party-pooper person. My name is Martie, and I usually introduce myself to strangers as Martie Party – which is funny, I think, because the only parties I go to are family celebrations. I need to be with people who know me and my restrictions.

Being resilient is accepting reality and getting on with it. If you cannot play your favorite sport, then watch someone else. I was fortunate my first knee replacement was in 2003 when Roger Federer won his first Wimbledon. As much as I loved tennis, in the past I rarely had time to watch it because of the demands of a busy household – single mother, remember. I am so very grateful I could watch this amazing man until the day he retired. Even though I could no longer play, I could still enjoy the game and it transported me out of my bedroom.

I found this with horses, as well, I could watch them and love them knowing I will never be on one again.

Life changes and resilience is all about accepting that change.

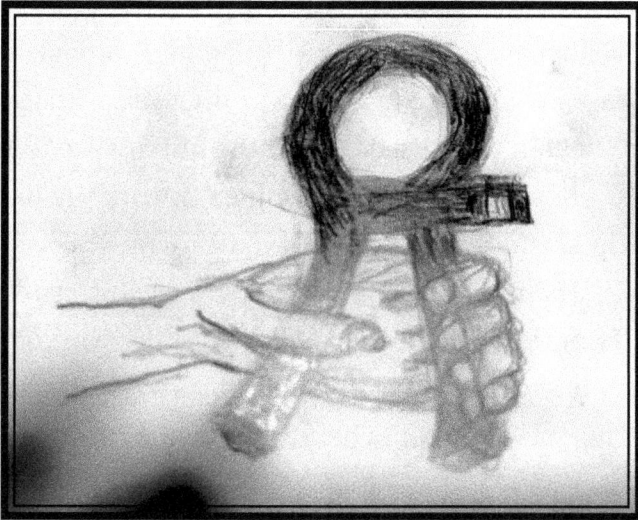

ROUTINE

Routine and regimen are often confused. A medical regimen is a treatment plan, but routine is what it will take to implement that plan.

When I have been rehabbing after every surgery or injury, I established a routine. In fact, it is a routine that will help you when your brain goes fuzzy with pain because the routine will be imprinted and will help you stick to the plan.

Every night, I have a basic routine which encompasses caring for my eyes, my weak hands, breathing through an apparatus to help my nighttime breathing, doing shoulder exercises for both shoulders, and attending to whatever miscellaneous body part is cranky, like stretching my IT band or hip flexors.

Besides the usual rituals of brushing my teeth, cleaning and moisturizing my skin, I always cover my eyes with an eye pad I have pre-heated for 30 seconds in the microwave. Whilst that is perched on my head for five minutes, I work my hands with a hand grip strengthener, I have two of them which I call Pete and Repeat. If I have had a bad day or something hasn't gone my way and I am upset, I put more vigor into the workout. I press out the bad energy shooting invisible darts to my annoyances of the day. This has helped my hands and is the reason I can type this manuscript.

I have macular degeneration, so the eye treatments are critical for my eyesight. The oil glands in my eyes get activated and keep the fluid juicy and flowing.

I take extra care of my teeth because for about 10 years I was having surgery after surgery and joint replacements galore, so I could not safely go to a dentist because of possible contamination from the decay in my mouth, to the joints in whichever part I'd had replaced. I never really figured that out, but trust me, there is a lot I haven't figured out about disability and the human body.

I also use a BREATHER to help with sleep. I had been diagnosed with sleep apnea, but the machines had been so annoying and painful, they were no help. In despair, I found a YouTube channel and learned about the Breather. It transformed my sleep. I think I still snore but gone are the wake-up interruptions I endured for about 10 years – I was always being awakened by pain, so the sleep apnea wasn't the primary focus of my medical needs.

The last thing I do before I go to sleep is to give gratitude for my day. Even if it has been a painful one, I believe it will be temporary and tomorrow will be a better day. I give thanks to the miracle of modern medicine for all the replaced joints and diminished pain. I know I am so much luckier than the aunt who had this challenge. Her only future was a wheelchair, and for me I realize I am so lucky that a wheelchair is a temporary conveyance when going long distances, like airports.

Those are my nighttime routines. My most cherished daylight routine is waking up, making a pot of decaffeinated coffee, doing a Bridge class on the computer, then going to the pool at least 3 times, and sometimes 4 times a week. Two days a week I participate in an arthritis class sponsored by the Arthritis Association. It is fulfilling for me to think of a connection with the Arthritis Association because I reached out in the past to see if they were interested in the story I am telling you now, but I never got a return call. I'm thinking mine is a story they hear over and over several times a day.

My other cherished daily routines are to take care of my house plants and my outside garden plants. Also, meal prep is a situation I take very seriously. I have quirky dietary needs such as needing gluten-free, dairy-free, and low-carb meals.

I am a nightmare to invite to dinner. Fine by me, because

eating alone is not a hardship. I often prefer it. Of course, when my family is around, we get each other's food regimens and there aren't any issues. Explaining why I am a gluten-free, dairy-free, flexitarian gets tiresome, so I try to stick to my own meal plans.

SELF CARE

I have touched on this subject all through this book. You must learn to be your own advocate and take care of yourself.

Of course, if you cannot drive, walk, or read, it gets complicated. I live in a 55+ golf cart friendly community, so I can get out to the pool, the bank, drug store and grocery store.

Driving is a sacred privilege to some of my fellow elders. They cannot conceive of the loss of freedom and independence the car gives them. I find this terrifying on some level, because the reflexes of an 80-year-old are no longer in quick response mode. Fortunately, this is a community of very little traffic where elders and younger people acknowledge the idiosyncrasies of their fellow citizens.

I had to give up driving in 2014 when I was 66 years old. A cervical fusion made my neck stiff and unbending, so I can only look straight ahead. Safe to say, I have tunnel vision and can only peripherally see oncoming traffic, which makes me an unsafe driver of a car. Therefore, I drive a golf cart named Tootsie. We only go 14 mph, but it is freedom. I can get to most of the places I need to go by myself. I cherish my independence.

For doctor's appointments, I am lucky to live in a community that has volunteer drivers. Honestly, it is a gift beyond measure for me. I average about 4-6 doctor appointments a month and the cost of taking an Uber became prohibitive. I am so grateful for these gentle volunteers.

The loss of mobility is the hardest skill to reclaim. Crutches, walkers, scooters, wheelchairs, braces, and canes are all aides to get you out and back in the game, but none of them are particularly easy. The world is not accommodating to us hobbler people, and it can be exhausting trying to keep up with a mobile life.

For me, I make myself walk whenever I can. It was about 10 years before I could find my stride because every time I got up, another surgery came along and knocked me down. My spinal surgeon wanted me to walk a mile a day, of course with a walker. I did this. I needed one of my daughters to take me to a park. Mobile phones now have step-counters so you know if you've gone a mile. Enduring painful step after a painful step was agonizing and there were many times I wanted to give up.

For a visual idea of what I was doing, I looked pretty dorky with my walker circling a playground where children were playing. The children in their loose and flexible bodies reminded me I was not always trapped by my disease, I had the gift of a very vigorous athletic life. Because I could no longer be that person didn't mean I had to stay at home in my easy chair and moan about things. The nice thing about walking outdoors is that the air is full of positive energy – sunlight and nature's bounty. Of course, if you live in a cold climate without sun, you can still get out and move around, maybe around a mall or the kitchen? Shake out the cobwebs, take control of your own life. It isn't easy, but the important things in life rarely are.

Loss of reading is a bit trickier but there are workarounds. E-books and audio books are wonderful ways to escape, even if bedridden. The daily need to do business transactions is a bit more frustrating. I cannot read the blue writing on a phone or a computer. I can enlarge the smaller texts or get someone to help me decipher the message. Simple things like instructions to open objects or how to operate an appliance are quite lost to me.

Fortunately for me, I can YouTube the product and there will be an inevitable How-To tutorial. This has been a godsend to me – I have made mosaic tables, papier mache, cleaned clogged drains, replaced refrigerator filters, cured many an ache and pain, done chair yoga, gotten gardening advice – the opportunities to find information are endless with today's resources.

I find the most important aspect of self-care is how you speak to yourself. How you overcome the negativity of the situation – the pain, the isolation, can be improved by your determination to get better.

Hygiene and mental health are also critical aspects. Stinky people are often ostracized because of their smell. Staying clean is not easy. Especially if your bowels and bladder are in constant commotion.

My personal hygiene used to be something that I took for granted as I was mindlessly running out the door for whatever activity, it isn't that I was dirty or stinky, but it didn't consume so much of my time.

Nowadays, self-care consumes most of my day in a way it never did before. I am grateful to live in a clean and safe environment. I have no idea how homeless disabled people find a way. My heart reaches out to them.

For mental health, there is so much crossover between the physical and mental needs of a human being. We need to stay safe, and if you are struggling with a chronic illness or an acute injury, safety is first and foremost.

Pain can make you edgy and agitated and you want to flail about in agony. Trust me, I have been there. But in the flailing around part, please stay home and safe in bed because missteps and tantrums will make you extremely unstable, emotionally and physically.

Setting your mind to getting better – doing physical therapy, getting strength training – none of that is easy or comfortable, but it is extraordinarily important and probably the only way out of having cranky body parts control your life.

Having a healing environment can soothe your mind, having someone to talk to can soothe your soul. You are going to need help in your healing journey, both physically and emotionally.

I find mindfulness invaluable. I am constantly learning about it. I hope you can learn about it because it will ease your anxiety.

SLEEP

Let's get this straight, if you have a painful condition, sleeping will become your biggest challenge because pain wants you to suffer, not slumber.

If you have a severe pain problem, you will often wake up with sweat covering your entire body. It is so exhausting. You are wet, you are exhausted, and if you have a double bed and live alone like I do, you can switch to the other side of the bed to escape the soddy mess your bedsheets have become.

If you have a partner, you really don't want to importune them with another problem at night, because they have often been importuned enough during the day and need their rest. So, the couch might be your best place to transfer your sweat-soaked body (after you change your nightclothes).

After my first rotator cuff surgery, a very helpful nurse counselled me on how to get comfortable to sleep with a shoulder injury. She told me to actually sleep on a couch and prop myself up in a way I could not move, because even the slightest movement with a shoulder can wake you up. I was so grateful to her. I had to have 4 more shoulder surgeries, and I used her advice after every one.

Then there is the sleep apnea issue. I didn't know I had this until after my first spinal fusion. When I was in the ICU (intensive care unit) after surgery, I had a nurse sitting beside me 24-7. At one point I stopped breathing, and the nurse yelled at me, "Do you know you have sleep apnea?" In fact, I did not know this, and I am grateful for the heads up – because I live alone and am oblivious to my sleeping patterns, except that sleep was elusive and disruptive.

I knew I snored, but apnea is the actual stoppage of breathing and can really strain your heart and has the scary potential to stop you from breathing indefinitely. The hospital takes sleep apnea very seriously, thank goodness.

After about 6 months when I had healed some, I made an appointment at a sleep center. The first order of business is a sleep study. This is a truly disturbing test – you have electrodes all over your trunk and skull. You are told to sleep but cannot take any sleep aides like Benadryl. It wasn't fun, but I was there to get a report, not pass a test.

My test showed I had severe sleep apnea. I had no idea. I was given a c-pap machine. I faithfully used the obnoxious machine for one year. The doctor could tell I was compliant because there is a monitoring system in the machine. Unfortunately, after one year of faithful use, my apnea did not improve and my doctor washed her hands of me, which happily coincided with my departure from that town.

When I got to the new city, I got a new sleep doctor. Again, I did a sleep study in a frightfully cold environment. I slept with sweats and three blankets. Again, the study showed I had severe sleep apnea. My new sleep doctor gave me a b-pap machine which would fix the problem. It did not.

I used the machine faithfully as verified by the computer read out. The problem was the mask connected with an elastic in the back of my head between my ears. My spinal fusion was aggravated and I would wake up with migraines. My sleep doctor didn't deal with migraines so he showed little regard for my dilemma. Well, Covid hit, and I moved one more time.

Four years ago, I took my apnea into my own hands. I had a massage therapist who worked with Navy Seals. She told me that they used a didgeridoo to help retrain the throat muscles to prevent soldiers snoring and apnea. This makes sense, the Navy Seals need to sleep in unpredictable places. No snoring allowed.

Emboldened with this knowledge, I tried a didgeridoo, my kids gave me one for a birthday. They are cute, but super hard to blow into, maybe because I am 5 foot 2 inches tall and not so strong in my elderly years.

Frustrated and somewhat desperate, I consulted my favorite physical therapists on YouTube, called Bob and Brad. They helped me with stretching, rehabbing, and sleep apnea. The sleep apnea apparatus they demonstrated is called The Breather. It transformed my sleep. I am not sure if I still snore, but six hours of solid sleep is the minimum these days instead of the 2-4 hours I would habitually get, if I were lucky.

Personally, I find sleep critical. If you are wandering around sleep deprived as many chronic pain patients are, you are in an even more foggy place because your brain never got to take a break.

The salient factor about sleep is that it is restorative and necessary. Sleeping pills and other medically induced methods sometimes help, but for me, it is more than a self-care routine. Letting my brain know we are going to shut down the noise for some much-needed rest. This process of finding peaceful sleep took me about three years, after I had finished my tenure of seven surgeries in five years. I had to transform my mindset from fearing the lack of sleep would undo me, to learning I could master my mind and body and find rest. Some of us don't cross the finish line with sleep and are still locked in the struggle. I have been there, and I wish you well finding your own formula for a healthy night's rest.

———

SURVIVOR

When you are in the thick of battle, you must focus on the task at hand. The replaced limb, the twitchy misbehaving body part must be the acute point of focus. Until you get the condition you have into a less acute phase, you will not be able to ignite the new world order that your body has in store for you. Hopefully, you'll be back on the golf course, the tennis court, the bridge table, walking the beach, rocking the baby – whatever was your go-to happy place. But early days are all about survival, getting stronger, and staying positive.

Staying positive is the hallmark of a survivor. It is that "Little Engine that Could" moment. "I can, I can, I think I can."

If your disability is permanent, the hardest hurdle will be accepting you will never return to your former glory. You have a life sentence with disease and disability, so surviving is going to take some gumption and courage. The hero of your own movie, so to speak. Get creative. I try to make a game out of adapting. I try to see myself as a valiant ninja fighting the demon Arthur. Of course, we know who is going to win the war, but I will try to win every battle. Even when I am in high states of pain, I try to remind myself that this, too, shall pass.

If you are a pessimistic sort of person and prefer complaining instead of seizing the day, then I hope you have a way not to make the people around you miserable.

Because the key to survival is having a good support team. Every hospital, rehab, doctor's office, or treatment room has people who are trained to help you. Listen to them, don't go all Rambo and try to tell them what they are doing wrong because, trust me, if you follow the program you will get better. Just stay the course and stretch a little bit farther when you can move – a little bit everyday adds up to a whole lot in the end.

Surviving a chronic illness has a special flavor all its own. Overcoming pain that others can't identify with, and walking a path other people don't have to travel. Survival is a lonely business. Yes, you need a team who understands your condition, but at the end of the day, the gumption and drive have to come from you. The power within. Tap it.

T

TECHNOLOGY

Technology is a tricky space. I can't imagine how I'd feel so connected to my loved ones, but for me, and I trust I can speak for many in my age group, it is twitchy and rapid paced, when my aged sensibilities want predictable and steady. Technology is the hare, and I am the tortoise, but those analogies no longer work because we no longer live in that steady as you go world. Today's modern hare has hyper-speed. The poor tortoise doesn't have a chance.

I was born before television and cell phones and computers and the internet. My parents had mostly transportation challenges, but rarely technological ones. For me, it seems like my free time and good will are often sucked dry by some technological blip. The modem doesn't work, the portal the doctors want me to use is complicated and time consuming, the myriad of things that were once manual are now completed and complicated by machines.

I must say I do like being able to deposit a check on my phone and it is marvelous getting things delivered to my door, and being able to talk to my family in Europe for free when it used to cost a fortune. These are the things technology has brought me for which I am very grateful.

However, technology can be a real drag and time suck for someone with limited and impaired eyesight. I cannot read the blue print on computer screens, I cannot read the fine print, and because 7 surgeries in 5 years kept me out of the computer loop, I lost my ability to understand what is happening.

The thing about technology to me is that it is a rapid-fire event. So often whatever I am seeking pops up on the screen, and if I don't push or click quickly, it disappears. Of course, at my age, I blame the younger generation. It would be lovely if there was a play space for the tech-savvy types and a slo-mo space for the elderly.

Technology has taken over so many aspects of our lives, and I believe we are in a transition. Once us old fogies leave the planet, I am thinking there will be a great sigh of relief so the younger ones can zoom to new heights, a sentiment shared by many of my elderly friends. The technological scramble to comply with medical portals, test results, prescription refills – it truly boggles my mind and dampens my spirit.

TIME

I find it fascinating that when I am bedridden, I become hyper focused on time. I need a wall clock or some visible timepiece to feel at ease. I don't have appointments to keep, so it is an irrational need to witness the passage of time. Even though I am no longer a participant in daily life comings and goings, I recognize I am just a spectator. Nonetheless, I like to know the time.

I would think this is a weird fetish of mine, but I have witnessed this need in other patients. My brother, who was suffering with AIDS, wanted a clock by his side. This was 30 years ago, so cell phones and the personal assistant apps were not available. I often think of him when I can ask my AI helper what time it is, what's the weather outside, please play my favorite song.

I am reminded of the days when a turntable and stereo speakers ate up most of my college dorm room. Technology has obviously streamlined our existence, but are we happier for it? Some days I love technology, other days not so much.

Time waits for no one. And time is one tick at a time when you are bedridden. Sometimes I want time to hurry up so I can take a much-needed pain pill, or sometimes I want it to slow down. People are quirky and time is a constant. I think bedridden people want the connection with consistency.

TRAUMA

This has been the most challenging and emotional word to write about because it has had the most impact on my life. For a few days, I stopped writing and struggled with my own resistances, because trauma has altered the shape of my life and writing about it pulls me back in time, when I prefer to be in the present.

I have faced my fears for many years in therapy, so to bring them back into my consciousness was scary. I need to explain my experiences with trauma because it is a multi-layered event, which a lot of people don't understand unless they have personally experienced it.

Let's start with a definition of trauma because I believe this is one of the most misunderstood of concepts. Trauma, trauma, it's everywhere. The little-discussed issue is: what is it? AI overview tells me, "Trauma is a deeply distressing or overwhelming experience that can have a significant and lasting negative impact on a person's mental, emotional, and physical well-being. There is trauma from war, sexual abuse, domestic abuse, car accidents, random assaults, academic failures, financial problems, mental illness, chronic illness, pandemics, natural disasters, and add whatever trauma you're dealing with to the mix.

Trauma is divided into 3 categories: acute, chronic or complex.

Acute is from a single incident – like a car accident or a natural disaster.

Chronic is on-going and incessant, like domestic abuse or the ravages of a chronic illness.

Complex is the result of having a variety of multiple traumatic events. The soldier who walks away from the war is not going to have the same after-effects as someone disabled or paralyzed. The woman who ends up in a domestic shelter with three kids is not going to have the same trauma as someone in a rotten marriage who took the car keys and ran out the door. The severity of the events is a crucial definition.

Now, to go deeper, there are actually 5 responses to trauma: fight, flight, freeze, fawn, and fine.

Fight is the instinct to duke it out, to get the better of an opponent, but what if that opponent is not present? There is a tendency to want to pound out the anger. Sadly, family members are the witness to this rage.

Flight is the instinct to run away. Flee. Good idea if a hurricane is barreling toward you, but so many folks take flight from themselves and their loved ones. They escape. Diversion, distraction, addictions – those kinds of escapes.

Freeze is when your system shuts down. You become robotic in your mind and body. Not listening to valuable survival messages. Remember Freeze Tag? I have, personally, not really frozen in a disaster, but I have seen others stopped in their tracks. Immobile.

Fawn is the urge to appease and placate whatever force has created the stimuli for rage – making bargains, promises. This is my most prevalent response pattern. I will try to lighten any event with a joke. There is a term called "bright siding," I will try to find the light in dark and dangerous situations. Can be super annoying if over the top.

Fine is when you have stuffed it all in a lock box in your body, mind and spirit. Never to be opened. To pretend not to hurt or care, and it becomes another emotional robotic response like freezing, just with a more moveable aspect. Keeping calm and getting on works until the past trauma crawls into your psyche and your behavior becomes aberrant – withdrawing from loved ones, getting a bit too drunk too often, zoning out on weird websites. You get the picture. Because no matter how valiant and brave you were under fire, the aftereffects of that battle are in your psyche somewhere and remember, *The Body Keeps the Score.*

Ironically, I am familiar with all on the above list, although I have never been in a combat zone or military outfit. My husband, Bob, was drafted after college graduation in 1969. Bob had been roommates with a young man named Dennis who was the sole survivor of his marine unit trapped in a rice paddy in Vietnam. He had lost most of his right arm which was sad on so many levels, because he had held the state record for discus throwing.

Dennis was one of the kindest people I have ever met, but at night, the terrors would rage and Bob would try to talk him down from his nightmares. Sadly, it freaked out Bob to such an extent, he was certain he did not want to go to Vietnam which was reinforced by the absence of his friends at our wedding – they were all in Vietnam.

When Bob's draft notice came, he decided to enlist in the Air Force because he felt he would not be put in a combat zone. Remember at that time, there wasn't a volunteer army, it was conscripted young men who went to war. Many of them ill-suited for the rigors of combat, which described Bob perfectly. He had been offered an internship in an ad agency in New York City prior to graduation. Those opportunities vanished when he entered the Air Force.

I had no illusions this was going to go well. In high school, I read Stephen Crane's "Red Badge of Courage." It was a tale of a young man during the Civil War. What he endured convinced me that war is hell, add to that the pacifism of a Quaker household, and I was a born rebel.

When Bob enlisted in the Air Force, he had to commit to four years instead of the two he would have served in the Army. We were stationed in San Antonio, Texas, and lived in very meager circumstances, a half of a trailer parked in a giant parking lot complex with a wall air conditioner which rarely worked. Hmm. Not sure many of you have experienced a summer in a hot and humid area with no air conditioning, but it's necessary to become resourceful. I'd put our sheets in the freezer in the morning before I left for work at an oil refinery. The year was 1969, so I pray conditions have improved.

Later we moved to a REAL trailer park with some trees and grass instead of a parking lot. We were on the flight pattern for the "Nightingales," the term used for the planes bringing the war wounded to hospitals at Kelly and Lackland Air Force bases.

While I was awaiting the arrival of our baby, I was not able to work while pregnant in those days, so I was sequestered at home in the trailer, which had been upgraded to full size and had a swamp cooler, not much of an improvement. I found any excuse to be diverted, and watching the Nightingales fly in with their red crosses on their side was my obsessive observation and was truly depressing. So many planes, so many wounded. It always brought me back to the human casualties and legacies of war, and I would see the raw face of war during the delivery of my daughter which I described earlier in the book.

At the time, I was not afflicted with a chronic illness. I was able-bodied and able to teach fourth grade at the local school. Our lives had improved and we moved into a house in a neighborhood, but I'll never forget the Nightingales. Most of the houses in our neighborhood housed women and children as the men were away at war.

There is much to admire about the military – the organization, the efficiency. However, for me, it was the human casualty that was foremost in my mind at the time.

Bob changed during his years of service. It was a frenetic time – lots of demonstrating. Lots of unrest. If one does not have a strong mind, one can become lost. Bob got lost.

His rages and bouts of depression became unbearable, and I was so frustrated he would not seek help. A Priest (he was Catholic) during the "Chaplains call" recommended he leave the Air Force because he was obviously under great duress. Bob wouldn't hear of it. How I wish he had. I divorced him 3 years after leaving the Air Force because he couldn't seem to leave his demons behind.

Sexual abuse trauma is also on my trauma list. When I was 8 years old, 6 months before my mother died, I was enticed by a neighborhood boy to come into his bedroom. I didn't sense any danger, his mother and grandmother were there. The removal of clothes with a boy didn't really bother me because I played Doctor with my brother. It was when he pushed me down and started injecting things into my vagina that I screamed bloody murder, pushed him off me, and got dressed and ran away. As I was fleeing his house, his mother and grandmother were both sitting there with great sorrow on their faces. They had to have known, they had to have been too subjugated to protest.

As I talk about my weight gain the year my mother died. I believe this molest was what was lodged somewhere in my body. Of course, I didn't tell anyone. I think until the MeToo Movement, no one talked about it. Or the priests who molested children. Why aren't we all on a rampage about this? Molesting children is a vile form of animalism that I had prayed disappeared with the Cave Man. My disease didn't, and I guess predatory sexuality is also a disease.

On my first date in high school, it was the Junior Prom and I was just a sophomore going with an older guy (by one year). He picked me up in a limousine which should have been a red flag, the year was 1964, not many people went to proms in limos in those days. All went well at the dance, it was super fun. But on the ride home, in the back of that limousine, he tried to have his way with me, and I was so shocked, I just froze. I guess that was my freeze response. I finally pushed him off me, but I never went on another date in high school, and I have never been fond of proms or limousines since.

It would be many years later that I would develop an autoimmune disease. I believe the stress of losing my mother at a young age, having an alcoholic stepmother, being sexually molested, living in a wartime military zone, having a debilitating genetic disease – all these traumatic events exacerbated my arthritis.

Chronic illness has left me with the inability to take a long walk, the inability to read, the inability to paint, the inability to drive a car, the inability to engage in all the sports I love, the inability to live without pain. It's quite a connection I have with trauma, and I would like to explain the after-effects because trauma affects your body, mind, and soul like no other condition.

Everyday there is a natural disaster somewhere. Hurricanes, tsunamis, earthquakes, floods, volcanoes erupting, firestorms, and tidal waves. Right now, there are fires raging on the West Coast where thousands of peoples' lives are irrevocably changed. So let's check out the collateral damage – trauma.

The term PTSD (Post Traumatic Stress Disorder) became

a popular term after the returning Vietnam Veterans weren't the same as the Returning World War II veterans. A universal world war is not the same as a regional war. Therefore, when the returning Vets from World War II came home, they were greeted as conquering heroes, but had no means to process their traumatic events, and I believe we are living in the aftermath of that unresolved trauma, the source of many a domestic violence scenario, an untapped rage within the human heart that recognizes that war is violent and how do we process the aftermath of that violence? Unfortunately, the targets of release are often perpetrated on the most vulnerable, like children, elderly people, and disabled people.

To this day, Veterans have medical care for physical ailments incurred in battle, but there is a commensurate collision with untreated emotional trauma because of whatever war or conflict our country engages in to keep the peace.

We don't want emotionally compromised veterans. The term shell shocked was used after World War I, but was dropped from the public forum as World War II seemed inevitable. We don't want freaked out people going to battle, we want STRONG warriors, of both mind and body.

I recently watched a documentary where modern-day veterans from Iraq and Afghanistan are using psychedelics to heal. Very radical and unsanctioned by the FDA, so the veterans in the documentary I watched had to go to Mexico for treatment. This really gets my goat. Wouldn't you open any door to help the returning vets?

I get being a super power, I get that we need warriors to protect us from invasion, but what I don't get is why we don't treat those warriors with more respect, gratitude, and emotional support when they return.

Because this is where the body, mind, and spirit are the most poignant. One's body may have survived a conflict – a war, a rape, abuse, accident – but the mind won't let it go. The thought that you are not safe will circle through your mind with rumination, regret, re-examination – over and over again. There is a book called "The Body Keeps the Score" by Bessel van der Kolk, which helped me heal like no other book I have ever read, and which has been the go-to book for understanding the lasting effects of trauma.

I was taught as a child to shake things off. When my mother died when I was 8, I was not allowed to talk about her death. I was supposed to be quiet and accept my fate. I did that. I gained 50 pounds that year. Weight would become a barometer for my mental stress. Not necessarily because I overate, but because my body wouldn't process any nourishment. I was trapped in my own grief.

Enter an alcoholic stepmother when I was 9, and it was going to be a good long time before I could face the pain and trauma of that childhood.

My body didn't want to let go. My mind kept telling me it wasn't safe, so it was my spirit that helped me endure. As a child, I was valiantly independent. I rarely considered home a safe space, so I spent my time busy with taking care of my horse, sports, clubs, academics, and friends. I am grateful I had any friends at all because looking back I was a bit of a hot mess.

Truly, friends can connect you to yourself in a way a family can't, and for that I am extraordinarily grateful. When I see movies about children who have unresolved trauma, they are usually loners, not feeling comfortable to be part of the crowd. But for me, I was the opposite. Friends helped me shine. Their support made me somewhat popular, and it is lovely to feel appreciated, something I rarely got at home.

That childhood fear of abandonment and neglect never really goes away, it can soften and you can rationalize with yourself, but honestly, if I weren't writing this book I wouldn't have articulated what pain has cost me.

The wind is blowing as I write this. The wind has always unnerved me in unexplainable ways. I think it is a lingering hypervigilance from my own traumas. I know the wind does damage, at least where I live, and I know the wind can create hurricanes and firestorms, both of which I have evacuated from, and both of which carried devastation in their path. So, me being unnerved is somewhat rational, if inconvenient.

On the other hand, the 30 mile an hour wind blowing today is not a hurricane or a firestorm, but somehow my body remembers. It keeps the score, and my mind is the statistician that keeps me in that mindset. I have to put myself through some emotional gymnastics to really focus on the task at hand.

True healing has to come from the spirit, the will to get better and thrive. Think about it – when we die, our body is still here, when we lose our minds nobody knows where it goes (think Alzheimer's) but our body will still be here. The part of us that is truly alive and the essence of our being has left. Our spirit has joined the cosmos – and whatever your personal feelings about the afterlife are, I am hoping you can find comfort in nourishing your spirit while you are still breathing.

This is where a good therapist can be invaluable. I've counted up the number of years I have been in therapy on and off, the grand total is 20 years since I was 29, now I am 76 so the therapists have entered during specific traumas in my life. Two of those years were spent in analysis, where I went 4 times a week for an hour at a time. This was very expensive, but it was a cost I was willing to pay. I wanted to work through the twists and turns of my life so I would not visit my demons on my children. I probably did that anyway, but I know the impact was less severe because I faced my pain, I didn't numb it with substances, I didn't take up with an inappropriate partner or drain the family finances. I went to therapy.

I knew in my spirit and soul that I needed help to remind myself of my own humanity, my own goodness. I think this is what a good therapist can do for you. Lift you out of the black hole of misery and doubt that are the residue of trauma.

The problem with therapy is that it is expensive. I have never added up how much I spent on therapy because it was not a luxury, it was an essential.

Today, YouTube has some extraordinarily good counselors dispensing advice for free or at least the cost of the subscription.

I personally watch a website every day that has helped me through an incredibly complicated scenario with one of my troubled children. Mental illness is real, my friends. Not sure Trauma is considered a mental illness, but I am thinking PTSD and CPTSD (Complex Post Traumatic Stress Disorder) are real, and I believe they are finally getting the respect they deserve, instead of "keep calm, carry on" or "suck it up" – that sort of mantra. Those mantras have helped me in the midst of the struggle, but when the trauma subsides, its residue needs to be unpacked, not carried through years and lifetimes and generations.

U

UNDERWEAR

I, personally, had to give up wearing underwear about 10 years ago. It also gave up on me. No more fashionable bras for different outfits, in fact, no more bras at all. For you gentlemen out there, it may not be such a relevant subject, but some women are challenged with this. It isn't a political, feminist statement, it is a fact.

Between neck and shoulder and back surgeries, it dawned on me that bras were a thing of my personal past. It's a sense of indecency for some of us from a different generation. But trust me on this, when it happens to you, if it does, it is not an easy accommodation to make. Fortunately, I am old and was old when the necessity hit to go braless, because people aren't really checking you out anymore. It could also be because of the cane, the walker, the wheelchair – or whatever apparatus helps you navigate life, that clues people off to the fact you are different.

Braless-ness is different for different women and it definitely depends on the size of your breasts. Small breasted women might pay "no never mind" but for me, it is an obvious fact I face when dressing – are my boobs going to betray my disability? As if it is not already on parade, but it speaks to our sense of decorum and pride. For me, I often need an ever-trusty sports bra, but I couldn't put on a conventional bra because my hands cannot manipulate the closure mechanism, my back is full of metal cages supporting my spine. A metal clasp would send me into a painful episode. So, no bra.

The underpants part of underwear is probably universal between men and women. To put on a pair of underpants is not impossible for me, but it always takes some contorting and needing assistance from a grab bar, and sitting on a chair. I know a lady who uses her bathroom mirror at foot level to try to negotiate the putting one foot in the right slot – hoping you got it on the first try (rarely happens unless you have a grab bar apparatus at hand).

I have a spinal fusion so I cannot look down to see where my foot is going. I hate putting on sweat pants, bathing suits, under-wear, regular pants – or God forbid, stockings. This sounds silly unless you are in this predicament.

Therefore, I am uncouth. I go out into the world with no one aware I have no underwear. You know what? They don't care. Unless I'd just written about it for all the world to know, I don't think people notice because it truly is none of their business.

It is not un-hygienic and it is not morally reprehensible, but still it tends to be a cultural norm. I remember my younger years.

In 1978 when I started my company managing doctor's offices, I had to dress demurely in case I inflamed passions or seemed slutty. Because I needed to fit in with men I wore dull suits, but underneath, I had sexy panties and bras. I loved feeling feminine and didn't want to be a boring person in a boring suit sitting in boring meeting after boring meeting. Because I had a secret, I was not boring. I would not become mundane and transparent just to succeed. Of course, I was never transparent because I was quite often the only woman at the table. Little did they guess I had hot pants on under the boring pants. We must find a way to keep true to ourselves. I have never been a promiscuous sort of person. I like sex to be personal and private, so I felt very personal and private with my sexy underwear.

Those days disappeared about 12 surgeries ago. I cannot give you an exact date because I don't remember. But it was a sad transition. I wish I'd kept some to remind me of the glory days when my disease wasn't driving the bus.

URGENCY

This conjures up two types of urgency: the one to get to the bathroom ASAP, and the one to heal as fast as possible to get back in the game pronto.

The first one is tricky. Toileting becomes a complex space for a disabled person. So many places have a one- person-at-a-time scenario. This is a bit daunting if there are no grab bars or counters to hoist yourself up. The multi-plex places have handicapped spaces, but I find them so often occupied when I truly have an urgent need and cannot wait for the occupant to empty.

I once frequented a big name grocery store where one of the employees routinely changed her clothes in there. Oh ugh. One hates to pull the Disability Card and challenge, I have to go! If I end up in a regular space, I have nothing to leverage myself up. It took a lot of core training and hip flexing squats to be able to walk, but getting up from a toilet takes some space and a bit of support. I eventually figure a way out, but it is not the quick stop most able-bodied people experience.

Then there is the urgency to get back in the game, to be part of the scene you knew. If this urgency card is played too soon, it will backfire on you. Healing takes time, and honestly, none of us want to waste more, but by hurrying your healing, you can aggravate the work that has been done, and possibly create a new problem.

I know you fast movers want to stay in the fast lane, but for now, the slow lane is your friend. Don't press it.

I once had physical therapy after a shoulder surgery. The therapist shared a story of a man who had had a shoulder replaced, and thought he was good to go, so he tried to replace the engine on his car. Please do not try this. Take the time it takes to mend.

UTOPIA

We all have a vision of a perfect world. For Gladiators, it was the Greek Elysian Fields, "where the souls of the heroic and pure reside after death." I think that was a clever way to motivate people to fight to the death, but for me, I know there is no such place. Perhaps in the afterlife, but on this Earth, we must deal with the here and now. I do not believe in perfection. If we lived in such a universe, children would not be born with disabling genetic diseases, and there would be a goal worth fighting for besides money and fame.

And yet, I think people get stuck into believing their disability or ailment means they can never have joy again. Not true. Maybe they are in a freeze response stage and cannot see a way out of their misery.

For me, in the here and now, it would be a Utopian wonder if people stopped using disabled people's parking spaces, there were ramps and accessibility into every building, there was no pain so powerful to stop destroying people's lives and livelihood, and children were born into complete and stable environments.

On that last note about children. I have been so angry for a long time about the suffering of childhood. For many, it starts in the cradle. When I lived in a big metropolitan city, I used to take Ubers and Lyfts to my doctor's appointments. It was at least a half-hour to an hour ride, so I would strike up a conversation because I like people. I had to sit in the front seat because my neck wouldn't bend to put me in the back seat. It makes the separation of being in the back seat less of a conversational barrier.

As we were driving along, I would, in the course of conversation, not right off the bat, ask the driver this question. Pretend the entire earth is a virtual laboratory. Pretend there are only ten children born a year. I would hold up both hands – ten fingers. I would ask the driver how many of those children will be born into families that can accommodate their needs, the categories were emotional, financial, environmental, cultural, and physical. The answer was generally 1-3, and that was a quiz

I gave over about 2 years to more than 20 drivers. Perhaps if they were in a Rolls Royce, they'd offer a different answer, but that speaks to the divide between the HAVES and HAVENOTS, and is out of the scope of this book.

My personal take away was – as a world chock full of people, we are not doing a good job giving children a welcome to our planet.

V

VICTIM

The Cambridge Dictionary's definition of victim is "someone or something that has been hurt, damaged, or killed or has suffered, either because of the actions of someone or something else, or because of illness or chance."

We can all agree being a victim sucks. We can all understand that being killed is the ultimate form of victimhood. We can all understand this definition, I believe.

However, sometimes people work the victim card too long. It becomes their identity. I have been a victim of domestic abuse and a vicious disease, but I refuse to adopt the victim mentality. The belief in reciprocity, that the world needs to compensate for one's predicament is relative to the degree of severity of the circumstances. I have met people from the Holocaust who generally want to wake people up to the horror.

I knew one such valiant Holocaust survivor who went around to high schools to explain about hate and evil and war. One hopes they listened.

I get veterans feeling a certain rage at the treatment they receive upon return. I had a friend who had been a captain in the army during Vietnam. When he got out, he went to a Job Fair for Veterans in Washington D.C. The attitude as he described it to me was, "Ooh, you killed people, how can we trust you?"

My captain friend had to be one of the smartest people I ever knew, because he figured out that if he went to the Open Jobs Fair the next day and didn't report his military service, he would be hired. Because the year was 1970 with no computer checkpoints, he was hired, and eventually became vice president of a large, prestigious bank. Isn't that amazing? The very people we send to defend us during war are not trustworthy during peace?

I was a victim of domestic abuse. Not physical abuse, but extraordinary coercive control and emotional abuse. My second husband was an Axis II category of insane. Incurable. I tried to understand him, get therapy with him, protect me and my children from him, but nothing worked. One night when he was in his rage, we packed up and left.

In Family Court, he was the victim. His wife and family had abandoned him. It took me four years and a large portion of my financial resources to finally get the court to see his madness. That was after he had kidnapped my children to Mexico and abandoned them for 3 days. I was so grateful for their safe return, but now I had two very wounded teenaged children, who had to overcome a bloody nightmare in addition to coping with the transition to adulthood with a disabled mother.

How can I or any of us know this bizarre behavior exists unless we experience it? TV Shows and Lifetime movies rarely delve into this sort of insanity, or if they do and I missed it, I probably wouldn't watch because reality and fiction are miles apart and I don't want to relive the nightmare of that time.

Perhaps being labeled a VICTIM has never suited my self-image. Yes, I have had a devastating disease and a trauma-filled life, but I choose to live in the peace and beauty of NOW, not THEN. That peace of mind came with years of talk therapy. I am grateful I live in a safe community where I can find sanctuary and comfort.

If your tragedy has been indelibly written in your soul, then I feel very sad for you, because it is very important as Dylan Thomas wrote: "To rage against the Dying of the Light." He was talking about old age, but a disease or disfigurement can make one old before one's time.

To me, there are so many categories of victimhood – Holocaust survivors, wounded warriors, domestic abuse survivors, Black Lives Matter survivors, the MeToo movement survivors, but the survivor category that really makes me angry is children. We asked them into this world, so please try to stop making their lives so volatile. Get a grip on your demons.

VISION

My vision was compromised in 2005 when I took a drug I cannot name because I don't wish to fight the Big Pharma Lawyers. To my knowledge this drug is still advertised on television with the caveat "May cause blurred vision." Well, for me it caused a doozy of a problem. I couldn't read a regular book. Fortunately, e-books entered the scene and without that apparatus, I wouldn't be able to read at all.

The ability to see and read signposts is essential for survival. I always wear the blockout dark sunglasses like so many vision-impaired or blind people wear. Some folks clue in and help when I am stumbling to discern a sign or something, but if there aren't such helpful souls around, I am lost.

Because the multiple issue of loss of vision is the sensitivity to light, I literally cannot go outside without my glasses. It is enough to be hobbling and wielding my way through places, but when there are fluorescent lights, I am a wreck.

I recently went to the DMV (Department of Motor Vehicles) to renew my Handicapped Parking Placard. The wait was two hours regardless of a prior appointment.

I couldn't figure out why I was getting so nauseous and weak. Yes, the chairs were uncomfortable, but I got up and paced through the sea of people also waiting to relieve my back pain. Finally, when I got the placard in hand, and went outside, I realized I was fine because I had escaped the fluorescent lights.

This became a poignant issue for me because there are rooms and places I simply can't enter or stay in for long periods of time. For example, I had to give up playing Bridge because the fluorescent lights made me ill.

Many doctor's offices have fluorescent lighting. Often a very kind and understanding technician or doctor will turn off the overhead lights so I don't get nauseous. I am always so grateful for their kindness.

Most people don't care that I wear blackout glasses inside, but every now and then I will get a gib and I just laugh it off. I try to put on my "I am a rock star" attitude, but it stings. I wish tolerance were a more widespread phenomenon.

VULNERABLE

This cannot be stated enough. When you are in the throes of a disease or trauma, you are vulnerable in a way you have never experienced.

Refugees and evacuees and children and traumatized victims and old people are all vulnerable. But being disabled means you will always be vulnerable.

I rarely go to public places by myself. I stick to my home ground. Fortunately, I can drive a golf cart, but I am very aware that if I try to go off road and go Rambo, it will not go well.

I am grateful for my children and friends who understand and will still take me to lunch which is the height of my week. I was recently asked by a very kind gentleman to join him and his wife for a concert in a local restaurant. I had to decline. Restaurants for any long sit are not advisable and forget about the lighting issue. I usually attend restaurants that have comfortable chairs. You'd be surprised how many don't.

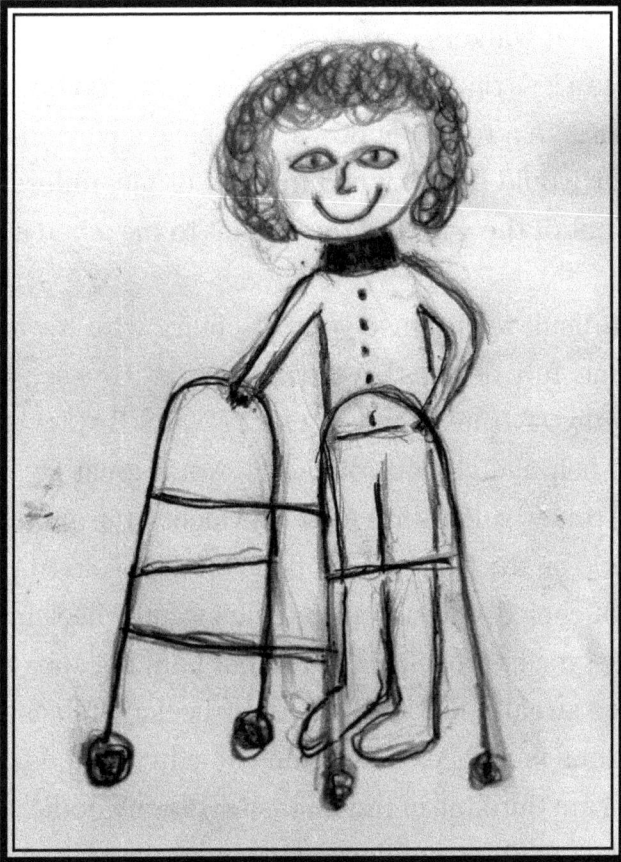

WALKERS

I am not talking about those people who are walking through the mall, or around an athletic field, or hikers, I am talking about that very clunky apparatus that helps people march through the world.

I have used a walker for many of my recoveries. Can't say I was greeted with joy when I entered a room of strangers. It is more likely I engendered an uncomfortable feeling. It does annoy me that walkers are so cumbersome and unfashionable.

Despite a less than welcoming reception, I could navigate my walker through a room, sit down, and have a conversation. But the walker would be stationed in front of me, unless someone moved it out of the way and returned it to me when it was time to leave.

It is difficult to disguise your disability with a walker. How about some fun designs? A little pizzazz? Greased Lightning would be my favorite. I had to use TENNIS BALLS on my last walker to help me glide through life. Not a great fashion statement. Old timey walkers are most prevalent – the aluminum ones with wheels on the front, tennis balls on the back. I'd love to see an array of choices in walkers and canes and wheelchairs. Actually, I see some improvement lately, but I am not sure how much these more streamlined walkers and wheelchairs cost. It would be marvelous if a wheelchair could come in all kinds of models, like cars. I am thinking of fun fantasies, like a Woodie or race car or chariot, something not depressing. Again, cost concerns.

Despite design and cost issues, some walkers have become more streamlined and light to manipulate. However, I still see way too many old-timey ones.

When you graduate to a cane, well, now that is a fine day because your prop is less conspicuous. Funny thing about canes, it is difficult to find a place to store them while you are sitting. You can put it on the ground, if you can bend to do so. Or you can hold it between your legs so it will be available when you're ready to go. It rarely hooks conveniently on the chair in front of you because it is a precarious position and can fall down which disables you if you have a back injury and cannot retrieve it. The stand-alone canes are a good idea, but too heavy for me to use. I have had five shoulder surgeries, and using a cane might help me walk steadier, but it would simultaneously stress out my shoulders and neck. So, I am free-wheeling these days. When I need to go long distances, I ride in a wheelchair if I am lucky enough to find someone to push me. I cannot use an electric wheelchair because I cannot turn my neck to see oncoming traffic. If I become more frail, I will invest in an electric wheelchair with massive mirrors so I don't plow into people.

WATER

Hydration is a modern fixation, I think, but with good reason. Water makes up almost 60% of an adult body and 78% of newborn babies.

I think it was almost 30 years ago when water became a THING – all of a sudden water bottles were showing up at the gym, the tennis courts, wherever athletic events were occurring.

Water should not be reserved for athletic endeavors. We must all work to become more hydrated, and water is the solution.

On the back of the bathroom door in the gym where I swim, there is a hydration chart. The more hydrated you are, the clearer your urine. The more yellowish, you need to take on more water.

The part that gets my goat is the plastic, single use water bottles purchased at the store. If that is all that is available, by all means use it. However, with deliberation and forward planning, one can use a water flask and have water on demand whenever one needs it. Some companies are even using logo-ed water bottles for their employees.

Sadly, I live in a community of elderly people who haven't gotten the memo about the toxicity of plastic. I am not an environmental harridan, but I do wish they would get the picture.

Funny thing is, I use a water bottle my daughter gave me with a picture of her dog. Before I brought that bottle to water exercise class, I was cajoled with comments like, "What's in the bottle, Martie? Tequila?" Now they ask about the dog. Sad to know there is such resistance in some communities about personal hydration and personal responsibility.

I think the problem for a lot of older people with drinking water is the need to visit the toilet more frequently. I would posit that if it makes you healthier to pee more, then what is the downside?

There are all manner of water substitutes – spritzes, coconut, sugar free fizzy drinks. Those can be a welcome break at times, but the main performer needs to be plain old water.

As a child, I once attended a camp where canteens were used for trail rides or long hikes. I thought that water tasted YUCKY, so I barely sipped from it. These days, I use filtered water from my refrigerator and I imbibe 6-8 glasses of water throughout the day. If I need to go shopping or be out for a long period of time, I bring my trusty flask. It is true that I have lost a few, but when the bottle is special, like with a picture of a beloved animal, I rarely forget it.

Spruce up your act, grab a water flask or canteen or a reusable plastic bottle, and start drinking!!!

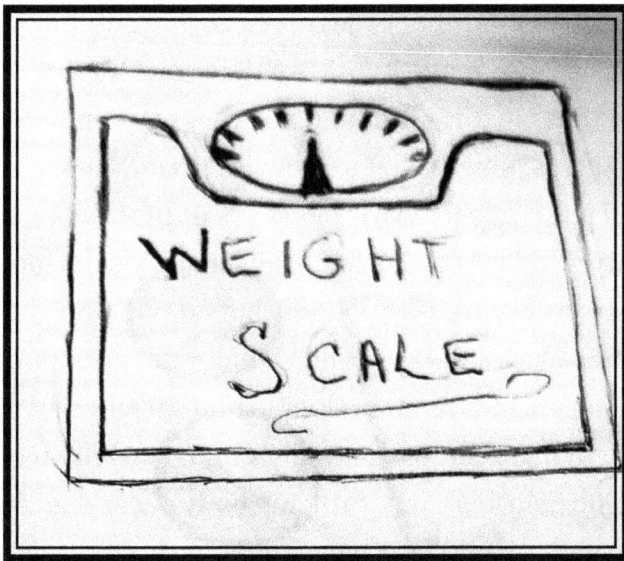

WEIGHT

This is a topic near and dear to my heart because weight gain and management has been the nemesis of my existence. Just looking at a scale sends shivers down my spine. I have tried to embrace the scale, tried to make friends with it, but it has been kryptonite to my self confidence.

I described the 50 pound weight gain when my mother died. As I grew, that weight gain became more distributed throughout my body, but I was still 20 or 30 pounds overweight. Fortunately, I was an athlete which helped it be more muscle than flab, but still made me very unfashionable in whatever costume I would wear – dresses, gym shorts, jeans, or bathing suits.

I spent a large majority of my time in athletic outfits, and yes, I was that big girl (although not very tall) that could hustle and make goals, sink baskets, or swim marathons.

When I left home to go to college, I lost the unwanted weight, which stayed away until I had children. Most women gained somewhere between 20-30 pounds, but not me – 35 with my first child and 55 with my last child. Mind you, I did eat unwisely with my first child – coconut donuts and green chili enchiladas were my cravings. But with my last child, I swam an hour a day and ate 2000 calories a day. Still, my body packed on 55 pounds.

That weight would be a permanent fixture for me with yoyo dieting and starving myself. Of course, there was that menopause weight gain that just wouldn't go away.

About 20 years ago, I got the memo about glutens, and that has been a godsend and has helped me keep the weight off.

What turned the page on this problem and finally helped me gain control of my weight was meeting a Canadian doctor who knew about Metabolic Resistance Syndrome, something I had never heard of. I wished I had heard of it, because I was that fat lady who ate well, but was trapped. Once I drank water for four days and gained 2 pounds, that is Metabolic Resistance Syndrome right there.

Under the auspices of the Canadian doctor, I ate 500 calories a day and I had daily injections of a hormone therapy drug. In one year, I lost 50 pounds – a pound a week. I stuck to this regime because I desperately wanted to reduce my body size. The weight wasn't healthy for my arthritis, but it also frightened me because I didn't want to be a hefty person my children would have to lift as my arthritis gnawed away at my body parts. I am so grateful to that doctor. I am so grateful I am in a body size that is manageable and liftable.

This is a very important topic, and I understand the frustrations many people face with weight loss. I think when people are newly disabled and homebound, the refrigerator has a siren's call of comfort.

My prayer is that people find a way to shed the pounds, they are not good for your heart or your joints or your self-esteem or your overall well-being. Nobody can do it for you. They can help you, like that kind doctor did for me, but you are the one in charge and I pray you find the willpower to reduce. Your body will thank you, your loved ones will thank you, and your life will be longer.

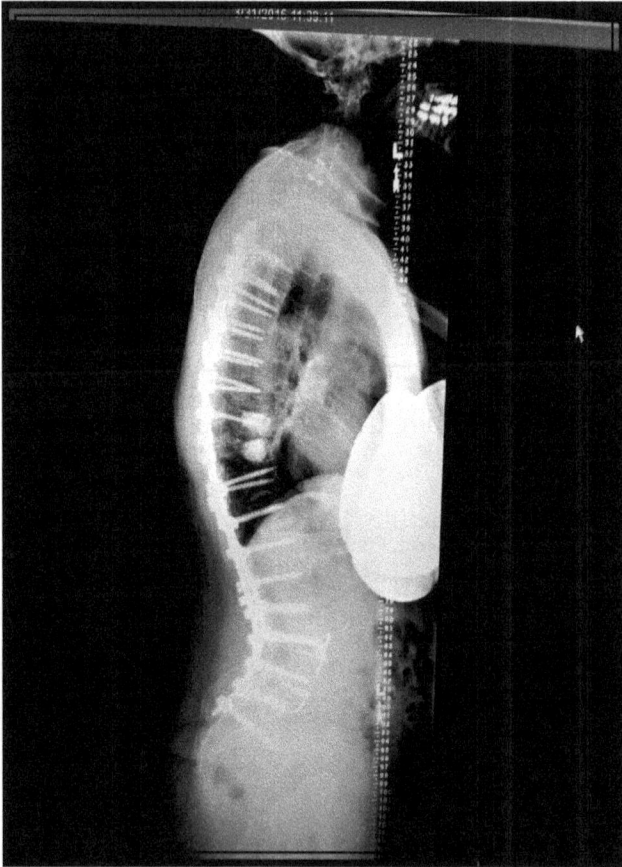

X-RAY

This is an x-ray of my spinal fusion. You can see that at every vertebrae there is a long screw, there are actually two of those at every level of my spine, even my neck (the neck x-ray isn't included because it's not as concise). It took 3 spinal surgeries to accomplish this fusion. Each of these surgeries were 8 hours or longer. I was asleep, but the surgical staff weren't. I imagine they knew how to give each other breaks, but I marvel at their stamina. When I thought of them taking that time to fix me, I tried to be as compliant as possible, which is a testament to my patience and their skill because I had, in total, 7 surgeries in 5 years.

After the first fusion, you feel every spike in your back. I called them "my forks" because I like to think I am funny and try to break the ice with humor, even if I am the only one in on the joke.

You can see why I almost named this book, "Full Metal Spine." I am hoping a picture is worth a thousand words because to describe the process would be tedious, but I will try.

My good fortune was that I had an amazing spinal surgeon. He was brave. He knew he could help me, and he did.

I think of him every day when I am able to walk around without the incessant pain of a crumbled back.

It required 3 separate surgeries. The first was from the sacrum to T-9. I was forewarned it would be a process that would require multiple surgeries.

That took 6 months to heal enough to try the next level. Unfortunately, the first fusion resulted in the rest of my back being broken, a condition my physician had forewarned me about. I walked around for six months with a broken back which is probably not the correct term, it was more like I had a crumbled spine above T-9. If a surgeon is reading this, please forgive my non exactness with medical terminology. After all, I was asleep.

When I meet the back complainers, and they are out there in groves, at first I try to explain what happened to me, but I give up because very few people listen to anything but their own problems. "Nobody knows the troubles I've seen," is their theme song, and I try to avoid people stuck in a rut.

The interesting thing about x-rays and me is that I now have metal knees, metal hips, metal spine, and one metal shoulder. Getting an MRI is not possible because of the amount of metal in me. I am okay with that because my mantra is NO MORE SURGERIES. I keep repeating that to my one non-metallic shoulder. I am so hopeful it listens because as much as I appreciate all the surgeries I have had, there comes a time for NO MORE.

Y

YES

This is one of the most important words for me to whisper to myself repeatedly. YES energy is positive and will help you on your road to healing.

Right after surgery or right after your accident, you will be laid low. But there are YES things you can do every day. Yes, you can sleep a little longer, feel a little better day by day. Maybe not today, but if you keep that YES in your head and see what positives come with each incremental improvement, you will make progress.

If you expect yourself to jump out of bed and regain your former movement or activities, then you are going to feel a loud NO! Because healing cannot be rushed. If you take every gain you make – a few more steps, a bit longer sitting up, an ability to keep something down in your roiling stomach, being able to dress yourself, and being able to toilet yourself. All these are massive gains in recovery, but if you are expecting the big recovery to happen in record time, think again. You are not trying to set speed records, you are trying to heal.

YES energy can turn your struggle into a resilient, defiant energy. It reminds me of the "I can, I can, I think I can" mantra of that little engine.

Like many elderly folks, I often walk into a room and forget why I went in there. There was a time I would berate myself, saying things to myself like, "How stupid" or, "How I hate being old", I would work myself into a bit of a chastised tizzy.

Since I adopted the YES way of being, I now walk into a room and if I've forgotten my purpose, I take a minute, take a few deep breaths, and I will say, "I knew I came in here for a reason. Please let me remember." And I generally do. It has become a game with me. Every time I recall what I was thinking and why I did something, instead of feeling like I lost a thread, I eventually remember, and I yell YES! And I give myself a mental gold star. It's turned a gap in memory into a victory of recall.

YOGA

I regret that I missed the yoga years. When I was younger, Jazzercize was the craze. It was the first time videos were available to work out at home. I loved it, but my joints did not because it was too aerobic.

In the beginning of the yoga years, I wanted to join and do conventional yoga, but I cannot sit in the lotus position or bend over and touch my toes. I tried one class and resigned myself that yoga was not for me.

Just recently, I discovered a chair yoga class with a lovely lady on YouTube. It truly is a remarkable practice for the mind, body, and spirit. It took a long time to find a space where I felt welcome but I am so grateful I did.

The breathing techniques can center your energy into your body. And stretching is beneficial to body and soul, plus the mind can take a break from worrying about whatever is going on in your life. Yoga can be a tremendous benefit to a healthy regimen. It hasn't always been my sentiment.

When I started walking with an obvious limp, I would have a fair amount of well-intentioned people say, "Have you tried yoga?" Politely, I would respond, "Thank you very much, but it is not an option for me." Rarely would they cease and desist their advice persisting with "it would be so good for you, etc., etc., etc."

Approaching a stranger (me) and suggesting yoga would heal me crossed so many boundaries – assumption of knowing my disease, assumption I hadn't tried it, assumption that they know exactly what I need to "fix" me.

This desire to fix strangers or to comment on their awkward gait grates on my nerves in an irrational way. I know they mean well, I know it seems right to them, but the presumption to diagnose and to prescribe something for a complete stranger is an invasion of personal privacy.

The underlying message is, "We want you to be like us, we don't want to see you limp." Now, this may not be their intention, but it has come to sit wrong with me. In the early years I was more tolerant of these comments. But there was a time when I'd see a yoga person coming with their mats and latex pants, I would turn the other way or cross the street.

I want to make a tee shirt that says, "Yes, I am disabled, but you didn't cause it, and I doubt you can fix it, and unless you're a physician of international renown who knows about degenerative joint disease, please keep your opinions to yourself." Of course, that is a tee shirt no one would read or produce. And people possibly would start to argue with me, "I was just trying to help."

Trying to help is the realm of good intentions gone awry. It probably sounds like I am being unkind about this, but I have been harangued and shamed by more than one yoga enthusiast, so I just steer clear of that space.

Interestingly, I couldn't do yoga, but I could do Pilates, which was invented by Joseph Pilates who had studied yoga and the movement of animals to help design the apparatuses he developed to help people.

I chose Pilates, and that rather quieted the yoga enthusiasts, because at least I was doing SOMETHING, right? Not just passively accepting my fate as if they knew what was happening to me.

When I lived in a community with my favorite Pilates teacher, I loved it. Now, I do not find that practice available, so I use water exercise as my go-to stretch and recovery space. The water is so buoyant. The joints that don't want to move on land will be weightless and compliant in the water.

So, no yoga for me, but I hope yoga, Pilates, water exercise, cycling, or hiking can engage your enthusiasm – something that fits your lifestyle so you can keep your body moving. I once met a woman at the gym who said, "Motion is the Lotion," it is what makes you feel juicy and alive.

Exercise is essential to health. We aren't meant to be couch potatoes, and we aren't meant to be sedentary. Try to find a way, and if it's yoga, then all the better.

YOUTH

When a young person is born with a disability, I feel anguish for them because I know they will have a life-long struggle to feel "normal". But I also have a simultaneous hope they will find a road to overcome, to be bold, to look people in the eye with confidence and courage.

A permanent disability at birth is a challenge I thankfully did not have to contend with, but there are other challenges for young people. Juvenile arthritis is real. It manifests with joint pain, swelling, loss of motion. The list is similar to adult arthritis and presents before the child is 16.

Essentially, in Juvenile Idiopathic Arthritis (JIA) the body's immune system mistakenly attacks some of its own healthy cells and tissue. Scientists don't know why this is so, but I am thinking it is unimaginable because besides extreme joint pain, the eyes, the skin, and the skeletal system are all affected.

Often, it goes into remission, never to return again, however, that is not a given and it requires a vigilant parent to insure the child gets the proper treatment. I am thinking that joint soreness is often a symptom of growing – the good old growing pains diagnosis, so it must be a complicated distinction.

However, for some kids, it truly is a bump in the road. When all your peers are bouncing into adulthood and you are stuck on the sidelines because your body just won't work right, it takes a brave heart to participate on any level.

My hope is that a compassionate adult helps the young person adapt so the stigma of disability doesn't persist. In fact, most juvenile arthritis is reversible, but I wanted to write about this because when people hear the word ARTHRITIS, they think of old people, but the young ones have it as well.

Z

ZEST

I am hoping as we hone in on the last letter of the alphabet and, if you have read this far, you get the major mission of this book is for you to find the ZEST in your life, even if it has thrown you a curveball.

Zest isn't a matter of motion, it is a matter of emotion. We can find energy and joy in so many ways. We can count our blessings instead of enumerating our hardships.

I am thinking you might be thinking, well, that's fine for you, because you are a glass half full sort of optimist, but even for you pessimists out there, I am thinking you can find a silver lining somewhere in your life. Mine that silver, expand that beauty, become BIG in your own life, not shrunken by your dilemma or disease.

Maybe it won't come easily. It took me 6 years after my last surgery to put this book together. Certainly, I had tried 3 previous times, but this time, I finally put the pieces together and voila – you are reading all about me.

For me, it is all about you. What are you going to do? How are you going to recover a smidgen of joy in your aching body? When are you going to shake off the bad thing that happened to you and find a path to discover the meaning and purpose of your life?

ZONE

Most athletes practice to get their body in condition to play whatever athletic endeavor they have chosen. This isn't just for professional athletes, because they weren't always pros and had to work their way up to whatever heights they have reached, the zone can be a place for anyone doing any endeavor.

Professional athletes are fun to watch, but I worry people surrender their own energy to live vicariously through others. I imagine most pros would admit they were given the gift of coordination, but were they given the gift of DRIVE – what it takes to succeed?

Runners talk about "hitting the wall", tennis players when they see the ball as big as a grapefruit, will tell you they are in the zone.

Getting in the zone takes practice. When I lost my ability to swim, a skill I had had since the age of 2 and one I could not do because of multiple shoulder and back surgeries, I decided to re-teach myself to swim. I was in my early 70's, but I did it. It took about 4 months to look like anything resembling my old strokes, but I did it. When I used to swim 70 lengths, now I swim 20, but those 20 are more precious to me than I can tell you, because it takes me back to when I was in the zone, when I could win race after race after race because I had practiced, and I had the will to prevail.

That is what I wish for you all – To find the will to prevail – yes, it is in there. Dormant, perhaps, so wake it up and get moving.

However, it is also a good idea to ZONE OUT sometimes. This becomes complicated when you are bedridden. Most of us will change rooms, go to a special place in the garden, but what if you are immobile and cannot leave your bed? Television can help numb the senses like nobody's business, but if you are like me, I get tired of the noise, the commercials, the endless ads for medications for diseases I have never heard of. My zone out is listening to podcasts and interviews of interesting people. If you listen to the lives of most notable people, you will hear that none of them, or few of them, had anything handed to them on a plate. They had to find a way. That is what I hope for you, Find a Way.

CONCLUSION

W riting this book is all about sharing my journey. My intention was to edify and explain the impact of my own story to dispel pre-conceived notions of disability. If you are disabled, I hope you see a fellow traveler, one who may not have your specific challenges, but one who never gave up.

The frustration and isolation of a debilitating disease can crush a person's spirit. That is where I want to bolster your resolve. It is the spirit that will help you survive. Your body may never be able to rebound, but your spirit can.

Going out, being social, being a part of a crowd, those are not scenes for me. I do play bridge and go to water exercise, but other than that, I find few social gatherings amenable to my needs. Sitting, interacting in social situations – these are very difficult because I cannot turn my head, so unless you are sitting right in front of me, I can't see you.

Writing this book made me feel less alone, as if there were a congregation of disabled people who might like to hear my story.

I also believe caregivers need to read this book, or at least expand their knowledge of what their patient is going through. It is one thing to take care of a patient's physical needs, but it would be lovely if the caregivers of the world (and I thank you all) could also understand the emotional quandary that is disability.

I tried to shed some light, I hope I did because I'd really like to change the stigma of disability to a validation and recognition of what a disabled person courageously endures daily.

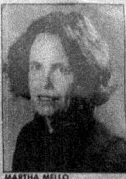

NEW RENO FIRM HELPS DOCTORS RUN THEIR OFFICES

By Rodney Foo, Journal staff writer

Nevada State Journal • Monday, November 30, 1981

I t's tough enough for a doctor to keep up with the latest medical journals, much less the newest Medicaid reimbursement rule.

Banking on the idea that a physician should be concentrating on medicine and not his accounts receivable, a fledgling firm—Physicians Management Systems—is taking aim at filling doctors' offices with their staffers.

In an age of specialization, PMS has found a niche that no other Reno firm has.

Quite simply, PMS hires and trains receptionists, book-keepers, insurance clerks, nurses and office managers to run the doctors' offices and process paperwork.

"The doctors we have love it because they don't have to worry about office staff." said Martha, an enterprising 33-year-old woman who started PMS two years ago.

"They just come in and they can have a good rapport with the staff because they are not the ones who are going to fire her. They're not the ones responsible for that. Once you take that barrier down you have a better working rapport."

"If there's a problem," said Kristin Haugen, 37, personnel director, "they call us."

But "problems" are the exception and not the rule, primarily because the firm takes care in its hiring practices, resulting in a low personnel turnover, they said.

"I can interview up to 50 people to find two who I feel are really qualified to do the job—which means in temperament, skill level and attitude," Haugen said.

"We look for an office complement of people that will fit together," she said. "Bright, intelligent people with certain cler-ical skills vs. 'I have had 20 years experience in bookkeeping or 20 years experience in Nursing.'

"We look for the total complement of the office. The people that work well together will provide better services for the doctor because his patients will be happier."

Interviews are held with clients to determine what they want and what type of office workers are best suited for their businesses, she said.

PMS pays its employees more than the usual rate, "We're

asking for intelligent, self-motivated people," Martha said. "Therefore, we want to reward them."

In addition, the firm offers their employees—who are on PMS' payroll—the opportunity for promotion as opposed to being a receptionist who works forever at that level.

"People in doctors' offices tend to get locked in dead-end jobs," Martha said. "For example, if you're a receptionist where do you have to go? In this company we have one girl who started as a receptionist a year-and-a-half ago. She's now going to be an office manager."

The women point out that an effectively managed office will increase the physician's cash flow.

We've walked into some offices where accounts were more than 120 days old and there was no charging for hospital bills, things like that, Martha said.

Martha, who worked at Saint Mary's Hospital medical staff department and did corporate work for its surgeons, started PMS after conducting a marketing survey as part of her business administration studies at the University of Nevada-Reno.

She concluded that "most doctors are overworked and I didn't feel they had the expertise or the time to deal with business matters" or the management of their offices.

"As a result, their offices are usually run inefficiently, which leads to an increase in medical care costs," she said.

Martha said some new doctors believe that once they set up practice, "My patients are going to pay me...The insurance companies will just send that money in."

"It just doesn't happen unless they know exactly what to do," she added.

And for a monthly fee and pay-roll costs, PMS will see to that problem and others, she said. The firm currently charges fees that range from $450 to $1,200.

Because the nurses and clerical personnel work for PMS and not the doctor's office, Martha and Haugen believe the system imparts a more professional attitude to the PMS employee.

"As communities become over doctored—and Reno is on the verge of that—there is more competition for patients and I think as you become more professional you can serve them better," Martha said.

Besides staffing and handling the paperwork for doctors, PMS also can help a doctor find a new office, redecorate it, or do consulting work to evaluate how well his office is being managed.

ACKNOWLEDGMENTS

I t truly takes a village to help a disabled person. I have been so lucky through this 47-year odyssey to have amazing help along the way. The only person there at the beginning was my first born, Katie. She was incredible. Only 7 years old, and she would massage my shoulders when we were on a long drive. She has been my North Star through this maze. I think my love for her was my guiding light through dark times before her sisters were born. Her sister, Alexa, is now also a Polaris, a never-moving beacon for me to find my way. But there were others along the way, and I have listed them in different categories – moral support, medical support, emotional support, financial and legal support.

MORAL SUPPORT

The moral support matrix I had through the years has changed players, but the core group has held fast. No words can encapsulate the gratitude, so naming them now will have to suffice.

Katie Cartiglia is my oldest daughter and has been with me the longest. She has also been living in Europe for the last thirty years, so her support wasn't always hands-on, but always precious. She came to help through more than a few surgeries and we try to have twice a year visits. Her presence is immeasurably important, and her love sustains me now that I am in my old age. We also make it a habit to connect every day via WhatsApp, the free internet service, to share our feelings and situations for unlimited talk time.

Alexa Gilweit is my youngest daughter, and I was also the youngest in my family. There is a saying that the youngest sometimes knows the parent the best. That has proven so true in our case. There is no one who knows how to help me and comfort me like she does. She lives in the same town, and she shows up in meaningful and significant ways. I know I wouldn't feel as safe living alone as I do with her present in my life. She is starting her own family now, and for her to have a life of joy and fulfillment enriches my faith that love is the greatest gift of all.

Charlie Cartiglia – my first-born grandchild. I was so lucky I was able-bodied when he was born. He and his sister remember me swimming and playing tennis and being bouncy and active. I am so grateful for you. Our talks keep me connected.

Lucia Cartiglia – My granddaughter who knows me so very well. Our visits, our laughs, are now superseded by her upcoming nuptials to a marvelous man. Her presence in my life adds so much light – like her namesake, only better.

Erik Harmuth is the husband of my daughter Alexa. Providence brought him to us, he is a strong and loyal partner to my daughter, and a strong and supportive addition to our family.

Samantha Malcolm who took me to many, many surgeries. We are no longer in contact, but I do cherish her.

Aurora Rueter doesn't remember our early years together.

She was born about the time I started having surgery after surgery. The blessing of her is that we had endless hours as Bed Buddies while I rested and recovered from many, many surgeries. You were and will always be, "my little love."

Gail Hammond – best friend for over 35 years. She and I were Single Mothers Against the World together. Our adventures when I was able-bodied are relished in my memory bank under Happy Times. So much laughter amidst so much pain. How did we do it? And still we text, we visit, we love and we support. That is what best friends are for.

Lali Mitchell – mentor teacher in graduate school who became God Mother to my children. She came to us when we were hiding in a cabin, afraid of my demented husband. Her courage and her commitment to us will always warm my memories.

Annie Johns – she has been there through terrifying times. During one of the most harrowing nights of my life when my children were kept away from me by a vengeful father, she organized a phone call to distract my mind from the disaster of a demented husband. A calm and steady friend who could make me laugh in the darkest hour. I have cherished our connection these last 35 years. And she still makes me laugh!

Doree Sitterly was right there by Annie's side with both their husbands during the call on the first Christmas Eve without my children. There are some things you just never forget, and that night was a turning point for me. I was not alone. Thank you, also, for all the doggie help, what a gift you have been to me and the girls.

Page and John Davis – two people I've lost touch with. They were incredibly supportive when I had to flee my house the night before a shoulder surgery (which is not the topic of this book), and it makes me sad I don't know how to catch up with them.

Miriam Thomas – how can I describe her courage and strength? She was a pillar for me to lean on when the world was crumbling around me. My husband had gone mad, and she was the sane voice who kept me tethered to the planet. She protected my children and I will honor her until the end of days.

Tracy Martin took the picture on the back of the book cover. She is an incredible friend, creator, and art teacher. We pop out for dinner together when I am craving French fries. She warms my heart and is a part of our family.

Peg Fisher came to my aid when I needed help to actualize this book. I had struggled for years trying to figure out a way to write and I concluded a desktop computer was the best answer. Because I had been out of the techie loop for many years, I was clueless how to activate a new computer, much less a printer. Enter Peg who enlisted the help of her husband Tom, and daughter Colleen to help. You are all witnessing the result. Thank you, Peg.

MEDICAL SUPPORT

Shane Burch, M.D., I dedicated this book to him because had he not suggested it, I would never have written it. He reconstructed my spine over a span of four years. I think of him every day with great fondness that the surgeries were a success. He altered the course of my pain-ridden life to a more mobile life.

Elayne Garber, M.D., my valiant and talented rheumatologist

with whom I meet once a month. She gave me hand-saving injections for a year from the free samples she got from the drug companies. I am typing, painting, and writing because I have the use of my hands. I will be forever grateful.

James Blasingame, M.D., performed 3 of my 17 surgeries. A more kindly physician I have never met. He even operated on my daughter. I have such fondness for his competence and character.

Timothy Dawson, M.D., was my first legitimate pain doctor whom I met in 2006, and what a wonderful source of information he turned out to be. No other pain doctor has been as helpful as he. No other pain doctor has been as personable as he. I appreciate when a doctor remembers me. I don't expect special attention, it is just nice to have a positive relationship.

Monica Moore, M.D., was the primary care doctor who recommended I get off glutens. She cared for my daughter when she was extremely ill. Kindness and compassion are her operating modes besides being incredibly intelligent.

Dr. Jeffrey Thompson was the miracle worker for me with his sound, magnetic, and chiropractic therapies. He was the one who told me Alternative Medicine had done all it could do, now I needed surgical intervention. His wisdom, warmth, compassion, and humor really helped ease the pain.

Andrew Kim, D.O., is my current pain doctor. I haven't known him very long, but I can tell he is a man whose head hasn't over run his heart. When I saw him for the first time, I needed an ablation. Also, I had arthritis in my jaw. He took care of the procedures to help me, and his office was the one who compassionately covered my last treatment.

Regina King, D.D.S., has been a trustworthy and competent

dentist. I couldn't see a dentist for about 6 years because of surgery after surgery. She understood the problem. One time I went into her office in too much pain to properly lie down on the dental chair to get my teeth cleaned. She had the hygienist clean my teeth sitting up. Thank you.

PHYSICAL THERAPY

Jim Weathers is the massage therapist who traveled with the golf pros. I haven't seen him in 20 years, but I remember very well his competency and compassionate advice. I just googled him to see where he is and I came across an August 9, 2007, New York Times article about his travels with professional golfers. He has a fascinating story you can check out. I recommend it.

Nicola Cimino was my Pilates teacher extraordinaire. He and his husband, Lucien, also became dear friends. If we were walking around town, he would walk in front of me and I would put my hand on his shoulder. It was such a logical way to get around, single file. Not to mention my sessions with him helped my musculature be strong so the surgeries I endured had a quicker rehab time.

WanWan Mancini has been my massage therapist for four years. She comes to my house because I can't drive to get to her. She has the magic touch with her hands, her hot stones, and her strong competent treatments. Her husband, Jon, also helps me carry heavy things and takes my garbage cans out. Volunteering to help an old lady really lightens the load of my life.

Joshua Craig is a new addition to my wellbeing team. He is

a Rolfer who also practices Cranial Sacral therapy. He helped my jaw relax and open up from a surgery I had 7 years ago, who knew? I look forward to seeing him every week.

MENTAL HEALTH

Leah Smith is a therapist like no other I have met in my years of therapy and graduate school. She and I have never met in person, but she Skyped with me for over a span of four years. She was the person who directed me to read "The Body Keeps the Score." Somatically trained, she was a godsend through one of the roughest times of my life. She kept me grounded and I know my current mental healthiness is a result of her wise counsel.

Pam Flowerday is a psychic healer. She wrote a book called, "Ask Yourself, Understand and Unlock Your Psychic Power for Personal & Planetary Healing." I met her years ago when I was going through an extraordinary personal crisis. Talking to her was like opening a window in my spirit that I didn't realize was closed. She also gave me great counsel when I thought of writing this book.

LEGAL AND FINANCIAL

Joslin Davis orchestrated an incredibly difficult legal problem when I needed to divorce my very demented second husband. I needed to protect my children, and she was extraordinary. When I think of the risks she took on our behalf, I am so indebted to her courage. Madness is a scary proposition in any human, but in a court procedure, it is not so obvious who is telling the truth. I am so grateful for her competence and compassion.

Tom Seidel has been my financial manager for almost 40 years. He has been through all my surgeries, traumas, and location moves. He has kept my money safe and secure, something so very rare these days, to completely trust who is managing the money.

Filippo Cartiglia, PhD, is a world-class economist who happens to be my son-in-law. He met my daughter her first week of college in 1989, and they have been a beautiful couple since. His financial guidance I respect, but his true treasure is being an excellent husband and father.

Dan Anaya was my insurance agent from the time I was in my early 30's. His advice and guidance through the maze that is insurance aided me time and time again.

Karen Hamilton, CPA, entered my life when the IRS decided to freeze my assets because I sold a property in Mexico. It was a really scary time for me. She guided me through many months of living in fear I had lost everything. Eventually, the mess was cleared up, and I got my money back with interest. I'll never forget her steadfast concern.

Larry Tannenbaum, attorney at law, is the husband of my best friend Gail, and has given me advice throughout the years. He connected me to Karen Hamilton, helped me debunk a bogus bank claim, and is always willing to help. The best part of him, he makes my best friend very happy.

PUBLISHING TEAM

And last, but not least, is the publishing team who has had my back through pain episode after pain episode.

Tamira Luc is the circus master and publisher of DelucsLife. She is the admirable organizer of the team.

Monalisa Gutierrez is the guide who shepherded me during all the endless tech problems a 76 year-old non-computer savvy old lady stumbled through. She always starts her texts with "How are you feeling today?" I love that.

Kirstin Baron who is also a gentle assistant. I could not have finished this book without their gentle support. Thank you for your forbearance and trust during this process.

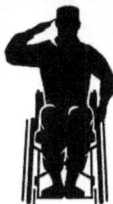

I n March of this year, I was invited to meet with the Paralyzed Veterans. Tam, my publisher, and I went to their location. I, myself, was quite anxious about this meeting. Here I had written a book about being disabled by disease, but these veterans were disabled by their service to our country. My worry was that I was a pacifist and they were warriors. Acceptance, for me, is often tenuous. Their generosity in receiving me and their willingness to include me in their circle touched my heart in unimaginable ways. Regardless of how we got there, it was understood that we were all on the same playing field now. We were all challenged by the adjustments disability demands. Their courage inspired me. One soldier had served in the 9/11 tragedy. The sights and situations these valiant men and women encounter daily humbled me. I was so grateful for their generous acceptance.

ABOUT THE AUTHOR

Martie McBride's life is a testament to her expertise in pain relief and management for individuals with chronic pain and disabilities. Having lived with degenerative joint discase for 47 years, she has experienced the many challenges that come with a disability. She has learned the most effective ways to manage her pain and continue thriving despite the limitations of her condition. Now in her 70s, Martie is dedicated to writing a book sharing everything she has learned from her journey while advocating for the rights of people with disabilities across the United States.

www.ingramcontent.com/pod-product-compliance
Lightning Source LLC
Chambersburg PA
CBHW070031100426
42740CB00013B/2659